the**facts**

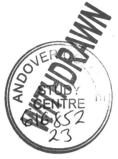

Panic
disorder

THIRD EDITION

STANLEY RACHMAN
Department of Psychology,
University of British Columbia,
Vancouver, Canada
and

†PADMAL DE SILVA
Institute of Psychiatry, King's College,
University of London
South London and Maudsley
National Health Service Trust, London

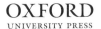

OXFORD
UNIVERSITY PRESS

OXFORD

UNIVERSITY PRESS

Great Clarendon Street, Oxford OX2 6DP

Oxford University Press is a department of the University of Oxford.
It furthers the University's objective of excellence in research, scholarship,
and education by publishing worldwide in

Oxford New York

Auckland Cape Town Dar es Salaam Hong Kong Karachi
Kuala Lumpur Madrid Melbourne Mexico City Nairobi
New Delhi Shanghai Taipei Toronto

With offices in

Argentina Austria Brazil Chile Czech Republic France Greece
Guatemala Hungary Italy Japan Poland Portugal Singapore
South Korea Switzerland Thailand Turkey Ukraine Vietnam

Oxford is a registered trade mark of Oxford University Press
in the UK and in certain other countries

Published in the United States
by Oxford University Press Inc., New York

© Oxford University Press 2010

The moral rights of the authors have been asserted
Database right Oxford University Press (maker)

First edition published 1996

Second edition published 2004

Third edition published 2010

British Library Cataloguing in Publication Data

Rachman, Stanley.
  Panic disorder / Stanley Rachman, Padmal de Silva. -- 3rd ed.
    p. cm. -- (The facts)
  ISBN 978-0-19-957469-8
  1. Panic disorders. I. De Silva, Padmal. II. Title.
  RC535.R267 2009
  616.85'223--dc22

                                2009024762

Typeset in Plantin
by Cepha Imaging Pvt. Ltd., Bangalore, India
Printed in Great Britain on acid-free paper by Ashford Colour Press Ltd, Gosport, Hampshire

ISBN 978-0-19-9574-698

10 9 8 7 6 5 4 3 2 1

Whilst every effort has been made to ensure that the contents of this book are as complete, accurate and
up-to-date as possible at the date of writing, Oxford University Press is not able to give any guarantee or
assurance that such is the case. Readers are urged to take appropriately qualified medical advice in all
cases. The information in this book is intended to be useful to the general reader, but should not be used
as a means of self-diagnosis or for the prescription of medication.

the**facts**

Panic
disorder

Also available in the**facts** series

Preface

This book is intended to provide the reader with basic information about panic disorder, which is relatively common. In our clinical practice we have found the need for a reliable book to recommend to sufferers and their families and friends. We hope that this book will also be of interest to the general reader.

In a major development the Department of Health is massively expanding access to psychological treatment for anxiety disorders, including panic disorder. The plan is to train 8000 new psychological therapists to provide evidence-based treatments, and reduce the lengthy waiting times, from 18 months to a few weeks. This progressive advance is extremely welcome news for sufferers and their families.

There has been much theoretical and clinical interest in panic disorder in the last few years, and we have tried to summarize this, and its relevance to patients today. In this edition, we have included up-to-date information based on recent work. We also give practical advice. References are provided for readers who may wish to read more widely. Research into panic disorder is continuing, and we await new developments and new findings.

S. R., *Vancouver*

September 2009

Foreword

I have read this book from a personal as well as a professional point of view. I know how terrifying the symptoms can be, having experienced panic disorder myself, and it is not something that I would trivialise.

During the last 15 years I have worked with anxiety sufferers at No Panic and the majority of our help-line callers phone because they are desperately afraid of panic attacks. They cannot believe such intense feelings of terror are not the precursor to a major mental/physical disaster. To get some sense of the scale of the problem, the No Panic charity took 75,000 calls to the help-line last year; imagine how immense the numbers of panic sufferers must be worldwide.

This book will be of great help to professionals and sufferers alike as it is extremely comprehensive and covers every aspect of the illness. The case studies illuminate the idiosyncrasies and false presumptions that sufferers begin to believe are realities. These mistaken beliefs are contradicted by the explanations given to patients to show how wrong their thinking processes are and how they can be changed, allowing progress towards recovery.

The chapter *Theories of panic disorder* is especially interesting as it shows how the illness has been approached over a period of years and both biological and psychological theories are covered by the authors.

I was delighted to see that the suggested treatments were practical, based on common sense, and compatible with what No Panic, as a self-help organisation, advocates.

It gives me great pleasure to be able to recommend this book; I think it will become an important contribution to the understanding of complex anxiety disorders.

Margaret Hawkins

Chairperson, NO PANIC

July 2009

Foreword

As cardiologists the manifestations and clinical consequences of panic disorders are commonly seen in our clinics. Having trained both as a cardiologist and general practitioner I am fully aware that the anxiety and uncertainty generated by both the initial attack and subsequent investigations cause sufferers further tension and anxiety and that the need for empathetic reassurance and, importantly, practical, concise, and understandable information about the condition and the potential treatment strategies available are paramount. This edition of *Panic Disorders, The Facts*, written by experts in the field provides simple, easy-to-understand and practical information and advice for both patients and healthcare professionals alike. The case vignettes will be readily recognised by those who have suffered from panic disorder and I believe both they and their clinicians will find reassurance in this well-balanced and practical publication.

Ed Nicol MD MRCP RAF

July 2009

Acknowledgements

We wish to express our gratitude to Gail Millard and Dona de Silva for their excellent secretarial help, and Michelle Moulds and Roz Shafran for their assistance in finding some key information. We are grateful to the staff of the Oxford University Press who gave valuable editorial advice at various stages. We also thank the authors and publishers who kindly permitted us to quote from their publications.

Contents

Introduction

Important developments have taken place since the second edition of this book was published in 2004. In October 2007, the Secretary of Health announced a massive expansion of psychological services for people suffering from anxiety disorders, such as panic disorder, and/or depression. The UK Government has embarked on a 6-year programme 'to provide better support for people with problems ... such as anxiety and depression', and approximately £170 million was allocated for the first three years. 'Psychological therapies have proved to be as effective as drugs in tackling these common mental health problems and often are more effective in the long run.' The aim is to 'reduce the average waiting time for psychological treatment from the current 18 months to a few weeks ... as the service rolls out'.

In order to achieve this goal '8000 newly-trained psychological therapists giving evidence-based treatment' are to be introduced (www.gnn.gov.uk—the government news network, article dated 10 October 2007). A related development was the publication of specific recommendations for treatment set out by the National Institute of Health and Clinical Excellence (NICE), an independent review organization that carries out comprehensive, regular evaluations of the available evidence. The NICE recommendations for treating panic disorders, and associated agoraphobia, are incorporated in this third edition. The insistence on using evidence-based treatments is an important advance. Unusually for an Institute of this type, the NICE recommendations also include clear statements about treatments that are not supported by acceptable evidence, and hence are not recommended.

In explaining to a senior engineer the new insistence on using only evidence-based psychological treatments, he asked: 'What were they based on before?'.

A considerable amount of research into the nature and treatment of anxiety disorders, such as panic, has been carried out over the past few years. Most of the research was designed to evaluate the effectiveness of psychological and pharmacological treatments, and the results are referred to in the present edition. Research into the nature and causes of anxiety disorders has not been neglected, and the major findings are integrated into the appropriate chapters.

Following the new style of this series of books, the key points are set out at the beginning of each chapter, and common questions about panic disorders are dealt with in the concluding chapter.

1

Panic and panic disorder

Key Points

- Panic disorders are psychological disorders.

- The main features of the disorder are repeated episodes of panic—abrupt episodes of intense fear, bordering on terror.

- The person fears an impending catastrophe, such as a heart attack.

- The episodes are accompanied by distressing bodily sensations, such as a pounding heart, shortness of breath, faintness, shaking.

- A proportion of the episodes are unexpected and inexplicable.

- The episodes generally last between 10 and 20 minutes.

- The episodes leave a residue of anxiety and the person feels shaken, exhausted, and emotionally drained.

- Recurrent episodes of panic often are followed by the development of extensive avoidance behaviour, such as crowded places, shopping alone, driving, bridges and tunnels, or even of being alone at home.

- Not infrequently the affected people experience a panic if they enter these situations ('situational panics').

- Their fear of having a panic in their dreaded situations can become pervasive, and in extreme cases they are housebound.

- Extensive avoidance behaviour, formerly called 'agoraphobia', can also develop without prior episodes of panic.

- Panic disorders are one of several forms of anxiety disorder (such as obsessive-compulsive disorders, post-traumatic disorders, acute stress disorders, intense health anxiety).

- Panic disorder is a treatable disorder.

What is panic?

A panic is an episode of intense fear of abrupt onset, usually peaking within a minute. The fear, often bordering on terror, is generally accompanied by unpleasant bodily sensations, difficulty in reasoning, and a feeling of imminent catastrophe: 'Something terrible is happening to me'; 'I am in great danger'.

The term 'panic' is derived from the name of the Greek god Pan. According to Greek mythology, the cloven-footed, dwarfish Pan was a lonely and moody god with an impish sense of humour who played practical jokes on humans. If a wanderer happened to pass the cave where he was hiding, Pan would jump out with a shrill and terrifying scream. The acute terror felt by the wanderers who experienced this treatment came to be called 'panic'.

Most people experience the occasional panic but if it is understandable and does not recur, no problems develop. However, a panic that occurs unexpectedly and inexplicably can give rise to a secondary fear. During the initial panic the person is likely to fear an imminent heart attack, choking, suffocation, or other serious threat. If the appropriate medical examinations reveal that the person is healthy and the feared threat to their safety is discounted, they are extremely relieved. However, if they then experience a second or third episode of panic, another fear arises. People are puzzled and alarmed by the recurrence of panics because they have been assured that their fears of a medical catastrophe are unfounded but they are experiencing repeated episodes of terror. The original fear, say of an imminent heart attack, is replaced by an intense fear of having panics.

 Case study

A 23-year-old woman described her first, unexpected episode of panic: 'I was at home one weekend and suddenly had trouble with my breathing. My heart was pounding and I began sweating heavily. I thought that my heart had given in and felt I was about to die. My husband rushed me to the hospital emergency where they tested my heart and assured me that there was no danger. I gradually calmed down and returned home after an hour or so feeling shaken but no longer terrified'. When she began to experience panics repeatedly it became evident that she had a significant psychological problem, and received psychological treatment.

Case study

A physically active security guard aged 32 experienced his first panic while exercising in a gym. During his usual exercise programme he suddenly became extremely worried about his rapid heartbeats; he felt that they signalled an imminent heart attack. Understandably, he became frightened and, gasping for air, asked a friend to call for an ambulance. He was rushed to the emergency room of the local hospital, and was frightened that he might die before reaching help. He was immediately wheeled into the examination room on arrival. No evidence of any cardiac irregularity or other problem was found, and he was assured that he was healthy and could return home, which he did after resting at the hospital for an hour. Two weeks later he had another unexpected panic while jogging, and again the doctors at the hospital reassured him about his health. A full examination carried out by his family doctor on the following day led to the diagnosis of a panic disorder, and he was referred for psychological treatment.

 Case study

A 26-year-old woman had a serious car accident while driving with her young child. Although neither was injured, she was very upset by the event. Several weeks later, she had a severe panic attack while driving on her own, and had to pull off the road; she could not continue with her journey. She was terrified by this, her first attack, which was followed by other frequent panics while driving. By the time she was referred to a specialist service she had stopped driving altogether.

 Case study

A female student suddenly began to feel weak in a crowded lecture theatre. She thought she was going to faint, although she had never fainted before, and fearing that she might lose control, quickly found an exit and left the lecture theatre. She felt relieved once outside, but subsequently began to have similar panics in comparably crowded rooms. These situations made her think: 'I will faint', 'I am going to lose control'. When she was referred for help, she had stopped going to classes and other crowded places.

A majority of patients panic because they fear an imminent heart attack, but other health threats are also capable of producing a panic.

 Case study

A 44-year-old businessman was vulnerable to panics when he experienced a sharp penetrating headache accompanied by feelings of weakness in his arms or legs. Whenever he sensed a panic coming on, he rushed to the nearest restroom because he felt less threatened when on his own, and away from scrutiny. In the bathroom he always, and promptly, examined his face in the mirror, and this was a clue to his underlying fear. The purpose of checking the appearance of his face was to ensure that his facial muscles were not paralysed, but remained normal and symmetrical. He was frightened of losing facial muscle control and hence checked for reassurance. It turned out that his paternal uncle had suffered a stroke at an early age and was left with a disfiguring weakness of the right side of his face. It was a source of intense embarrassment and concern to the uncle and discomfort for our patient during his own childhood. He had been scared by his uncle's appearance and tried to avoid him. During his adult years the patient became increasingly worried that he too might suffer a stroke, and the combination of a penetrating headache plus a feeling of muscular weakness in his limbs, became a trigger for panic. He experienced recurrent images of his disfigured uncle.

 Case study

Another patient had two related fears: one that she might have a heart attack and the other that she might have a stroke. Her first episode of panic occurred in a store after a prolonged period of family stress. Her heart was pounding, her face flushed and she had to gasp for air. 'I felt that my head would split open.' At the emergency room of her closest hospital they reassured her about her heart and allowed her to rest for an hour before going home. The episodes were sometimes preceded by sinusitis or a blocked nose; she believed that pressure could build up in her head and cause a stroke. Her father died at an early age from a stroke.

Case study

For another patient, intense nausea was the most prominent sign of an impending panic. As a result she severely restricted her diet to only those foods or bland drinks that she could manage without vomiting. This in turn made it virtually impossible for her to eat in public or accept social invitations. 'I feel utterly nauseous, freezing cold, shaky, and my body shuts down. My mouth is so dry that I can barely eat. My friends probably think that I am a freak.'

 Case study

The panics of another patient were set off by a fear that he was about to choke 'to death'. 'For example, last night I woke up at 2 a.m., all stuffed up, couldn't exhale, gasping for breath'. A variety of foods and drinks appeared to 'close up my throat, anything with vinegar in it, so salads are completely out. If I try to drink water after vigorous exercising, I'm frightened of choking to death—it is like drowning on land!'. He had been fearful of choking on certain foods since nearly choking on a sandwich, part of which had lodged in his throat and had had to be removed at the emergency service at his local hospital. His first full panic episode occurred when he was driving on a busy road and began to experience difficulty breathing. He felt that he was about to lose control and cause a serious accident, so he pulled up as soon as possible. A full panic ensued and he was unable to resume the drive for two hours. He slowly returned to his home, choosing the quietest roads, even though it meant taking a lengthy, roundabout route. He gradually lost the ability to drive unaccompanied and avoided all highways, busy roads and peak traffic periods, even though he acknowledged that he was a safe and dependable driver with an accident-free record. He was extremely frightened that if his throat 'closed up' when he was driving he would lose control of the vehicle.

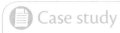 Case study

A young woman had her first panic after using a street drug at a party. It made her feel so strange, dizzy, de-personalized and out of control that she asked a friend to take her home as she was unable to find her way. She began to feel that she was going crazy and when she reached home, locked herself in her bedroom as she could not trust herself. The loss of control reminded her of a schoolfriend who had recently committed suicide by jumping off a high building, and was terrified that she might also kill herself. For a considerable period she continued to fear that she might lose control and as a result, restricted her activities and avoided being alone. Ultimately she was obliged to seek help and after a slow start made satisfactory progress during a course of cognitive behaviour therapy.

On average, episodes of panic last between 10 and 20 minutes, are extremely distressing, and leave the person feeling drained and apprehensive. Most people experience an occasional episode of panic in which the cause of the fear is evident. The threat of a serious motor accident can provoke it, as can an attack by a vicious dog, and so forth. These panics also are distressing and share some features of the unexpected panics, but at least they are easily understandable. In contrast, the episodes of panic that occur unexpectedly and for no clear reason are bewildering and, therefore, especially troubling. Panics that occur 'out of the blue', unpredictably and inexplicably, are a central feature of 'panic disorder'. The affected people begin to fear that they might be in danger of a cardiac arrest, or going crazy, or are hopelessly weak.

Some episodes of panic are predictable and the affected person takes steps to avoid the situations, places or activities that might trigger a panic. For example, a person who has an intense fear of contamination('I will contract AIDS if I touch a lavatory seat in a public toilet') anticipates that he will panic if he is obliged to use a public toilet. A person who fears suffocation might anticipate a panic if he is obliged to use a constricted stuffy elevator, a person who fears a heart attack might anticipate panicking in a supermarket. In instances of this type, called 'situational panics', the person tries to avoid the situations or activities that he believes are likely to precipitate a panic. This type of panic is partly predictable, and the expectation is sometimes confirmed, but in general the fear of experiencing one of these situational panics tends to be 'over-predicted'; that is, the person predicts far more panics than actually occur.

In cases of situational panic there usually is an underlying fear, such as a fear of contamination, that promotes the over-prediction of panics. 'If I go into that place or situation it will provoke an abrupt, intense burst of fear'. If the underlying fear is dealt with, then the dread of experiencing a situational panic fades.

It should be emphasized that most people experience occasional episodes of panic, which are not necessarily a sign of a psychological disorder. Experiencing an occasional episode of abrupt intense fear is common enough, and if it is understandable in the circumstances, such as a near-miss while driving in dangerous circumstances, it seldom has any adverse consequences.

(The term 'panic attacks' is commonly used but as these episodes of intense fear are not attacks, as in say 'heart attacks', we prefer to describe them as plain panics or episodes of panic. Ordinarily one does not speak of a fear attack.)

Panic disorder

In the widely used and comprehensive classification of psychological disorders set out by the American Psychiatric Association, the defining features of panic disorder are given as follows:

1. The person has repeatedly experienced unexpected episodes of panic.
2. In addition, at least one of the episodes was followed by persistent worries, lasting a month or more, of having another panic or by a significant change in the lifestyle or behaviour related to the panic attacks.
3. During the episodes, at least four of the following sensations/thoughts were experienced: pounding heart, shortness of breath, dizziness or faintness, increased heart rate, trembling or shaking, feeling of choking, sweating, stomach distress or nausea, feeling that one's surroundings or oneself are not quite real, feelings of numbness or tingling sensations, hot flushes or chills, chest pain or discomfort, a fear of dying, and a fear of losing control or of going crazy.
4. These attacks are not directly caused by a drug or a general medical condition.

In cases of panic disorder, the episodes may occur as often as daily or several times per week. After the first episode of unexpected, inexplicable panic, medical reassurance is usually sufficient to provide temporary relief and a sense of calm. However, when the second or subsequent episodes occur, conventional reassurance is of limited value. The person begins to fear that more episodes will take place and at unpredictable times and in any setting. He/she then becomes anxious and apprehensive and rarely achieves a satisfactory sense of safety.

The initial episode/s of panic tend to be unexpected, but as they recur, the person not only expects further episodes but is strongly inclined to over-predict the likelihood of further episodes. They also develop a kind of mental map of the potentially dangerous places or situations that must be avoided.

Panic disorder with agoraphobia

In a majority of cases, the occurrence of repeated panics is followed by restrictions of the person's regular activities. They avoid situations in which they fear that a panic might occur and/or situations from which a rapid escape might be difficult. These situations include supermarkets, theatres, cinemas, public transport, driving unaccompanied, bridges or tunnels, elevators, restaurants. Travel by underground train tends to be particularly worrying, as does being caught in a traffic jam or standing in a long line of people. In many instances the affected person becomes fearful even of being alone at home without the reassuring presence of a trusted person who can provide safety (such as by calling a doctor or an ambulance) if a catastrophe threatens. If these fears and the consequent avoidance of 'unsafe' places become excessive, the diagnosis of panic disorder is expanded to 'panic disorder with agoraphobia'. The term 'agoraphobia' strictly means 'fear of the marketplace' but is now generally used to refer to a fear of being in public places from which escape may be difficult.

Depending on the person's particular fears, the avoidance of 'unsafe' situations may be focused on one or a few places or, in severe cases, extend to virtually any place other than one's house, the company of a few trusted people, or hospitals. In these severe cases, the person becomes virtually housebound, unable to travel anywhere alone, and, even when accompanied by a trusted adult, can travel only short distances, using specific routes at specific times.

There is a close relation between episodes of panic and the development of agoraphobia but the connection between episodes of panic and a fear of being alone, even at home, can be overlooked. People who have an intense fear of experiencing a medical catastrophe, such as a stroke, or choking or suffocating, understandably try to ensure that help will be available. Their fear of being alone can be as intense and restricting as agoraphobia. They are inclined to anticipate a panic if they are left alone and/or help is not accessible. In these cases the person may refrain from travelling, especially to places that have limited medical services.

The persistent and unadaptive avoidance of certain public places or events can develop for reasons that do not arise from panics. Numbers of people who suffer from intense social anxiety, or who fear that they might lose control of their bodily functions, or lose control of their composure in public, or inadvertently spread contamination, are unadaptively avoidant of going out normally.

People who are extremely avoidant, with or without episodes of panic, often present a problem for therapists as they are unable to attend regularly and dependably.

Anxiety disorders

Panic disorder, with or without agoraphobia, is classified as a form of anxiety disorder, a broad category that includes all forms of psychological disorder in which anxiety is a central feature. The anxiety disorders include 'social phobias', in which the person experiences persistent anxiety in social situations, especially if exposed to the scrutiny of others, and 'specific phobias' in which the central feature is an extremely intense, persistent, circumscribed fear of a specific object or place (such as an extreme fear of spiders or heights). 'Obsessive–compulsive disorder' consists of repetitive, intentional, stereotyped acts such as compulsive handwashing, and/or repetitive, unwanted, intrusive thoughts of an unacceptable/repugnant quality which the affected person resists (see Rachman and de Silva 2009; see Appendix 5). 'Post-traumatic stress disorder' (PTSD) is characterized by intense fears that arise and persist after an unusually distressing experience such as a natural disaster, an accident, or a violent attack. The fears are accompanied by heightened levels of arousal, an involuntary tendency to recall or re-experience the event during dreams or at other times, and by strong tendencies to avoid people or places that are associated with the original stress. 'Generalized anxiety disorder' (GAD) is characterized by chronic, excessive, unrealistic anxiety about possible misfortunes, such as serious financial losses, ill-health, the welfare of one's children, or combinations of these misfortunes. Patients with this disorder are tense, restless, over-aroused, and over-vigilant. Their sleep is disturbed and as a result they frequently feel exceedingly tired.

The current classification of anxiety disorders does not yet include 'health anxiety', intense, unrealistic and unadaptive fears of having an illness and/or of contracting a serious illness. These fears were formerly classed as 'hypochondriasis', a term that implied exaggerated complaining and/or feigning, and it is fading out of use. The range of anxiety disorders is given in Table 1.1.

Mood disorders

Mood disorders are severe disturbances of mood that are persistent or recurrent. The main disorder is depression in which the person feels unremittingly sad and hopeless/helpless and experiences a number of accompanying bodily symptoms such as loss of energy, loss of weight, insomnia, and restlessness. Mania is diagnosed if the person experiences episodes of highly elevated mood, abnormal euphoria, over-activity, irritability, loss of judgement, etc. Some patients

Table 1.1 Anxiety disorders

Panic disorder, with or without agoraphobia.
Agoraphobia without a history of panics.
Social phobia.
Specific phobia.
Generalized anxiety disorder.
Obsessive–compulsive disorder.
Post-traumatic stress disorder.
Acute stress disorder.

have alternating depression and mania. They are diagnosed as suffering from bipolar mood disorder or manic–depressive disorder. Of the mood disorders, it is depression that is often found in those with panic disorder. Approximately one half to two-thirds of patients with panic disorder have concurrent depression; in roughly one-third of cases the depression precedes the panic disorder. The combination of depression and panic disorder is very debilitating. In some people the depression relates to the way in which the panic disorder interferes with one's life; in others, the depression is caused by factors unrelated to the panic disorder. The former type of depression tends to decline when the panic is treated; the latter often requires independent treatment.

A note on history

Panic disorder is not a new form of human experience. What is new is its recognition as a separate and identifiable psychological disorder. Although panic disorder was officially recognized as a separate psychiatric category only in 1980 (see Chapter 5), medical authorities had recognized and described panic attacks for a long time previously. The symptoms of panic disorder had been recognized in the past under various names including 'soldier's heart' and 'Da Costa's syndrome'. In a French medical text by Boissier de Sauvages published in 1752, he described intense anxiety states, including what he called 'panophobia'—severe shaking and feelings of terror. A British physician named Hope, in his textbook on cardiology published in 1832, wrote a clear and graphic description of panic, although the word 'panic' was not used. Since the middle of the nineteenth century, physicians have provided descriptions of patients who experienced panic, including many soldiers. Most of the panic patients were referred to cardiologists but the recognition that many of these symptoms had no physical basis, was slow to develop.

Treatment

As a result of a great deal of research and clinical investigations, two forms of treatment for panic disorder are now available: psychological therapy and/or medication. The details of these treatments, which are evidence-based, and recommended by the National Institute of Health and Clinical Excellence (NICE), are provided in Chapter 6. Panic disorder is a treatable disorder.

2

The experience of panic

Key Points

- Panics are episodes of intense fear during which the person has a sense of impending doom and dreads an imminent catastrophe.

- The fear is accompanied by a range of distressing bodily symptoms.

- The most common fears and distressing bodily symptoms are described.

- During a panic the person may feel trapped.

- Episodes of panic arise abruptly and are self-limiting.

- On average they last between 10 and 20 minutes.

- After a panic the person feels drained and anxious.

- Most sufferers develop a dread of future panics.

- They are inclined to develop extensive patterns of avoidance.

- Sufferers are inclined to avoid particular places/situations in which they fear a panic ('situational panics').

- Situational panics do occur but not as frequently as sufferers fear; they are over-predicted.

- Episodes of panic that come 'out of the blue' tend to be the most disruptive, puzzling and troubling.

- The first panic takes place in a public place (33%), while driving (25%), or at home (33%).

- Roughly one-quarter of sufferers from panic also experience occasional nocturnal panics.

- Nocturnal panics tend to occur early in the sleep cycle; the person awakes in a panic.

- They are similar to other panics and the person is conscious during the episode, and is able to recall it later.

The main features

Panic is a distressing episode of intense fear during which the person feels that a catastrophe is about to happen—they are having a heart attack or a stroke, losing all control, going insane, or losing consciousness. Although the average duration of a panic attack is between 10 and 20 minutes, at the time it seems to be endless. It is perfectly understandable to feel intensely frightened if you believe that you are about to die, which is a common thought in panic episodes. Moreover, the ability to reason is disrupted during panic. Patients say: 'My mind goes blank', 'I feel totally helpless', 'I can't think straight'. Facts that ordinarily would signify safety are difficult to recall or fail to provide the usual reassurance. For example, patients who experience tightness and pain in the chest interpret this as a sign of an impending heart attack, despite the fact that repeated medical tests have proved that their cardiac system is entirely normal. One patient said: 'At the time of the panic, I am *convinced* that my heart is giving in, even though at other times I know that I've repeatedly been given a clean bill of health'. The most common thoughts experienced during panic have been compiled by Dr Diane Chambless and her colleagues of the Temple University in Philadelphia, reproduced in Table 2.1. The thoughts are listed from the most commonly occurring thought to the least common.

Many physical sensations are associated with panic. The common and intense bodily sensations experienced during panic are listed in Table 2.2. Of these, the most common are: rapid heart beat, sweating, dizziness, shortness of breath and shaking; and the most intensely experienced sensations are: rapid heart beat, shaking, and shortness of breath. One patient had such intense sensations of a pounding heart that she sometimes felt her heart would actually burst right through her ribs! During one panic episode her heart rate was observed to

Table 2.1 Thoughts commonly experienced during panic

I will not be able to control myself.
I am going to act foolish.
I am going to pass out.
I am going to go crazy.
I will be paralysed by fear.
I will have a heart attack.
I am going to scream.
I am going to babble or talk funny.
I am going to have a stroke.
I am going to throw up.

From Chambless *et al.* (1984). See Appendix 5 for full reference. Reproduced with permission.

Table 2.2 Common bodily sensations experienced during panic

Rapid heart beat.
Dizziness.
Sweating.
Shortness of breath.
Shaking.
Hot or cold flushes.
Chest pain.
Faintness.
Choking.
Feelings of numbness.

From Barlow and Craske (1988). See Appendix 5 for full reference. Reproduced with permission.

increase by more than 25 beats per minute. It is not unusual to see an increase of 20 or more heart beats per minute during a panic (but in some episodes, little or no increase occurs). In a typical episode, people experience several of these bodily sensations, which increase in number during intense panics. In a really bad episode they can feel flooded by a rush of disturbing sensations, thereby intensifying the threat of losing control. The sensations are intrusive and they block calm and rational thinking about the true threat, if any exists. After being buffeted by these disturbing sensations and frightening thoughts, the person may be left anxious, shaken, even exhausted for between 30 minutes and several hours. Panics are self-limiting; they diminish spontaneously.

Episodes of panic leave a residue of anxiety. The person dreads a recurrence of the panic, and the possible loss of control during a panic (e.g. while driving). Moreover they are fearful and distressed by the absence of any reasonable explanation for these acute episodes of intense fear. It is not easily explicable and hence the panics are not predictable or controllable. In the circumstances many patients resort to avoidance; they try to keep away from situations/ activities that might provoke another panic.

Feeling trapped

During panics most people experience a feeling of being trapped, and their overwhelming thought and need is to escape. This powerful urge to flee can lead to impulsive, risky behaviour, such as driving too fast or recklessly, or dashing blindly out of a building. A patient who had experienced many panics became so apprehensive about panicking when driving her car that she began driving very slowly and only in the early or late hours of the day. Whenever she sensed the possible onset of a panic she stopped the car, regardless of the following traffic.

Experiences of this kind result in the avoidance of any similarly threatening situations. In the absence of any change in the occurrence of panics, patients keep adding to their list of places and situations to avoid, and in extreme cases become as housebound as people with major physical disabilities. Since they appear fit and healthy, their inability to leave the home can be puzzling to relatives and friends.

The first panic

Roughly one-third of the initial panics occur in public places, about one-quarter start while driving or being driven in a car, and one-third begin at home. In most cases it is possible to identify a major source of stress at, or shortly before, the first panic (such as personal conflicts, work stress, personal loss or grief, birth/pregnancy). The person's interpretation of, and reaction to, that first panic depends on the accompanying bodily sensations and the circumstances of the panic. A common example is an unexpected panic that features rapid heart beats, shortness of breath, and a sense of great danger. This is commonly interpreted as the start of a heart attack (or other medical catastrophe) and the person is taken to an emergency medical service. When the doctors conclude that the person's cardiac system is functioning normally, the person immediately feels relieved. However, it leaves unexplained the nature and cause of the discomfort and distress, and the absence of a satisfactory explanation is a breeding ground for anxiety.

When a second episode occurs and the doctors again confirm the absence of any cardiac or other medical problem, some patients begin to doubt their sanity. The episodes of anxiety are distressing and accompanied by intense bodily sensations that are undeniable and uncontrollable. But, so the reasoning goes, 'there is nothing medically wrong with me, yet I certainly am not imagining all this, nor making it up, and it is totally out of control. Am I perhaps going crazy?'. More accurately, the patient could conclude that there is nothing wrong with his/her cardiac system, but that they now have a problem of episodically uncontrollable anxiety—a problem as real and distressing as many physical problems. Regrettably, anxiety problems are less well understood, and hence less well tolerated by family, friends, and employers. Usually after the first panic, but certainly after subsequent panics, the person becomes extremely anxious and apprehensive. Additionally, he/she may become restless, irritable, and preoccupied with the problem. Once the person is persuaded by repeated medical reassurance that there is no danger of an imminent medical catastrophe, their anxiety may be focused on the danger of another panic. They begin to fear the panic itself—a fear of fear. Accordingly, when they anticipate having a panic they engage in strict avoidance of any places where a panic may be embarrassing or humiliating. The following case study illustrates this.

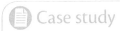 Case study

The first panic of Mr J, a 31-year-old shopkeeper, was provoked by a feeling of tightness in the chest accompanied by rapid breathing, which he took to mean that he was about to have a heart attack. After two more episodes, and extensive medical examinations, he was convinced that his health was, after all, sound. However, he now developed a fear of having panics, particularly as he felt out of control during those episodes. As a result he avoided driving or walking over bridges, driving on highways, and so forth, because he was frightened of having a panic, losing control of himself and causing an accident.

In many cases of panic disorder, the original fear of physical harm is replaced by a fear of loss of control or social embarrassment. Most often, the original fear is gradually replaced by the fear of having an episode of panic. For example: 'I dare not travel alone because I might have one of my panics'.

At the start of treatment, a detailed analysis of the first panic is of prime importance.

Unexpected panics

The most puzzling, and probably the most disruptive, panics are those that occur unexpectedly, 'out of the blue'. We have no trouble in understanding a panic that occurs in reaction to an obvious and predictable danger situation, such as encountering patches of black ice while driving in difficult conditions at night, but the panics that take place while sitting quietly at home are difficult to explain. There is no external threat and no reason to anticipate any threat, but with little warning the person begins to sweat, is short of breath, and has a pounding heart. Often these sensations are interpreted as signs of some internal threat, some danger to one's health. In the absence of any good explanation for the panic, it is virtually impossible to predict when and where the next episode will occur. The unpredictable and inexplicable qualities of these panics are an added worry and burden. As one cannot be fully assured of being safe at any time or place, it becomes difficult to plan activities. In the words of one patient, 'It is like an invisible enemy; it can occur wherever I am, whatever I am doing. But I can't see it or prepare for it. It has become an invisible threat'.

Some panics are triggered by frightening images. Intrusive 'pictures in the mind' can evoke a strong fear reaction and even a panic. A patient who observed her father die from a massive heart attack experienced recurrent images of the scene, and on occasions misinterpreted her shortness of breath and fast pulse as signs that she too was about to die suddenly. A patient who had been attacked during her teens had recurrent images of someone trying to strangle her, and when they intruded she inevitably felt acute fear. Certain disturbing intrusive images are remarkably persistent, and the content of the image tends to remain unchanged, even over many years. They also retain the power to evoke intense emotional reactions; in cases of panic the images usually evoke intense fear reactions. The images can be distressing and most patients strive to block them out, not always with success.

In the absence of clear signs of threat, sufferers tend to be guided by their moods. 'Yesterday I just knew that I daren't go out; I certainly would have panicked. I was uneasy and anxious from the moment I woke up.' In contrast, there are some days (which, alas, are fewer) on which the person feels calmly confident and knows that he/she is safe and unlikely to panic. Their plans for the day, going out or staying at home, are determined by these general feelings. Unfortunately we are all inclined to over-predict fear—we tend to predict that we will be more fearful under a given threat than turns out to be the case. A common example of this over-prediction occurs in anticipation of public speaking. For many people, the actual event turns out to be less fearful than they expected. Because of this broad tendency to over-predict one's fears, people with panic disorder are inclined to be significantly more avoidant than is warranted by their actual experiences of panic. They anticipate very many more panics than they actually experience.

With repeated episodes, it is possible to identify triggers for the unexpected panics, and detect some pattern in their occurrence. As will be seen in Chapter 4, the psychological consequences of unexpected panics are more serious and disruptive than those that follow predictable panics.

The occurrence of at least some unexpected panics is regarded as a diagnostic sign of a panic disorder.

Situational panics

Most panics occur in response to some perceived external threat, such as being enclosed in a small room. These situational panics share most of the features of unexpected panics, but are more predictable, and hence easier to avoid, than the unexpected variety. Situational panics tend to occur directly on exposure to the threatening situation, but the response is occasionally delayed. Strong anticipation of such an exposure can also cause a panic. Situational panics occur in virtually all cases of panic disorder, and are also common in most of the other anxiety disorders.

Nocturnal panics

Some people who experience episodes of panic are also affected by occasional panics during the early hours of sleep. Typically, the person wakes up in a state of panic. Studies suggest that about one-third of people with panic disorder have had this experience some nocturnal panics. Nocturnal panics share most of the characteristics of ordinary panics, including rapid heart beats and shortness of breath, plus rather more sensations of choking. In roughly half of nocturnal panics, patients report that their first symptom upon waking is a fearful thought, such as dying or losing control, and in the remaining half, the first symptom is a bodily sensation, such as choking. Nocturnal panics tend to be severe and last for roughly 25 minutes on average, although the duration can vary. Some people report very brief nocturnal panic attacks, lasting for one or two minutes, while others report a long duration. Nocturnal panics do not appear to be triggered by bad dreams, and unlike some other nocturnal disorders, panics are not accompanied by any disturbance of consciousness. During a nocturnal panic the person is normally responsive and attentive, and later can recall the event without difficulty.

Over half of all patients report at least one nocturnal panic, and up to one-third report frequent nocturnal panics. They are especially common among severe cases of panic disorder.

The exact cause of nocturnal panics is unclear. Some clinicians attribute them to respiratory disturbances, which wake the patient in a state of dread; but there is little evidence of respiratory disturbances in laboratory investigations of patients with panic disorder. Dr Michelle Craske of the University of California has suggested that nocturnal panics can occur if patients feel so threatened by possible catastrophes that they remain in a constant state of high vigilance. So, for example, patients who were particularly disturbed by an earthquake experienced fearful awakenings in response to subtle vibrations. Parents of sick children, and spouses and relatives of sick persons, are on high vigilance and easily respond, fearfully, to signs or sounds of discomfort in the ailing person. Such processing of sounds, vibrations and so on continues during sleep.

Patients who believe that they need to remain vigilant for signs of potential physical or mental harm to themselves or people close to them, feel uneasy if they begin to relax their attention, or fall asleep, during periods of threat. This accounts for the curious fact that some patients are so fearful of lowering their vigilance that they react anxiously to relaxation therapy.

The potential threats of harm, to themselves, tend to arise from certain bodily sensations that they associate with catastrophe and panic; mostly these are the same as the sensations that provoke daytime panics such as a pounding heart, shortness of breath, etc. These disturbing sensations are impossible to subdue at will and are inescapable, unlike places or situations that are recognized to be the sources of the threat and panic (e.g. supermarkets, buses). When the disturbing sensations, such as choking, occur in the confines of one's bed, there is no avoidance and no escape. Fortunately these fearful episodes diminish spontaneously, as do episodes of full panic. They are self-limiting.

Relaxation-induced panics

In most circumstances fear and relaxation have opposite effects and, as a result, relaxation techniques are a valuable and widely used means of reducing or blocking fear. However, in a small number of panic cases, the onset of relaxation actually triggers a panic. A 25-year-old who had experienced a bad reaction to a 'street' drug, which made her feel that she was drifting out of control, possibly to her death, developed a fear and avoidance of medications. She also had a panicky reaction to relaxation training because the spreading sensations of muscle relaxation re-evoked the sense of losing control and the threat of death.

These relaxation-induced panics generally arise from an intense fear of losing control and a consequent need to remain on high vigilance. In attempting to relax, their attention is drawn to bodily sensations about which they are already anxious; a further possibility is that relaxation reduces normal barriers to worrisome thoughts. Patients who tend to have panics during relaxation require a modified form of conventional treatment that excludes relaxation training unless special care is taken to overcome the person's reaction. In such cases, techniques of relaxation focusing more on imagery may be used.

3
Facts about panic

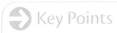 Key Points

- Many people experience occasional episodes of panic; this is not a sign of a psychological disorder.

- In most instances the fear is explicable in the circumstances, e.g. near misses.

- There is an association between panic disorder and agoraphobia.

- There is an association between panic disorder and depression.

- Episodes of panic are common in cases of anxiety disorder; most of them are secondary to the main problem, such as a fear of contamination.

- Most of these panics are situational and broadly predictable.

- When the primary problem of the anxiety disorder is treated the episodes of panic decline.

- Panic disorders can be precipitated by stress, loss, grief, increased responsibility, disturbed personal relationships.

- The risk factors for panic disorders include a sensitivity to anxiety, medical problems (such as respiratory illnesses), alcohol/drug abuse, use of street drugs, family conflicts, genetic factors.

- Approximately 15 out of 1000 people will experience panic disorder at some time in their life.

- The disorder tends to develop in early adulthood.

- There are rare cases of panic disorder in children.

- In most studies the disorder was found to be more common among women.

- If moderate to severe cases of panic disorder are not treated the problem can become chronic.

Frequency

Many people experience the occasional panic, without adverse or long-term consequences, particularly if the episode can be explained by an identifiable external threat, and is not unexpected. They have more difficulty coping with panics that come 'out of the blue', hence the importance that clinicians attach to severe, unexpected panics. Among the general population, up to one-third of people report having had at least one panic in the past year, but these panics tend to be less severe, as well as less frequent, than those associated with panic disorder. Having an occasional episode of panic is common and not a sign of any psychological disorder.

Panic and agoraphobia

Panic with agoraphobia is the combination of distressing episodes of sudden, intense fear, and the disabling avoidance of particular places/activities. It is unusual for agoraphobia to develop in the absence of a history of panics, but it does occur, and this is recognized in diagnostic schemes (see Table 1.1).

The most common consequence of repeated panics is the apprehensive avoidance of places or activities that have become associated with panic. People also tend to avoid situations from which easy, rapid escape might be difficult in the event of a panic (such as sitting in the centre row of a theatre, travelling by underground train). Agoraphobia was originally believed to be a fear of open spaces, but the fear and avoidance are generally more extensive than this. Prior to the introduction of the diagnosis of panic disorder, most patients who feared and avoided public and other places were given the diagnosis of agoraphobia and episodes of panic were regarded as incidental. The places usually avoided in agoraphobia are public transport, enclosed spaces, such as tunnels, bridges, slowed traffic, supermarkets, queues, and travelling long distances from home. Various activities, such as vigorous exercise or drinking coffee, can provoke anxiety, and are therefore avoided.

When a person is unable to avoid an anxiety-arousing place or situation, as in an unexpected traffic jam, he/she feels trapped and experiences an overwhelming urge to leave, to flee.

With their mobility and activities restricted, affected people are obliged to make numerous changes in their daily lives. Most sufferers find that the restrictions are eased somewhat when they are accompanied by a trusted adult; they can travel a little further (e.g. do the shopping, if accompanied). Patients who are taking tranquillizing medications generally feel that their mobility is slightly expanded when they are medicated. There is also some variation in their mobility, dependent on mood: on a 'good' day the person may be able to use a bus, but on a 'bad' day have difficulty even leaving the house.

Agoraphobia usually wanes when the episodes of panic cease or diminish.

Depression

There is an association between panic disorder and depression. Many sufferers from panic are also burdened with depression. It remains unclear whether the panic disorder generates symptoms of clinical depression, or whether the presence of depression makes a person vulnerable to panics. It is likely that the interaction can operate in either direction. Struggling to manage one's life when experiencing recurrent panics, and the consequent limitations on freedom of movement, is bound to be a miserable and demoralizing burden. Equally, a person who is labouring to cope despite feeling chronically miserable and hopeless, will be prone to make catastrophic interpretations of potential threats and of adverse changes in their bodily sensations.

Panic episodes in other anxiety disorders

Many people experience the occasional panic, but episodes are common among people suffering from one of the various forms of anxiety disorder—obsessional compulsive disorders, post-traumatic stress disorders, social phobias, driving phobias, specific phobias. In most instances, however, their episodes of panic do not 'come out of the blue'. They are situationally-linked. The affected people know that they might have a panic in specifiable circumstances; they are not unpredictable. For example, patients with an intense fear of contamination know full well that if they encounter a contaminated item or place (such as something dirty in a public lavatory) they are very likely to panic. Someone with a fear of driving over bridges knows that there is a possibility of panicking on the approach to a bridge, and so forth. The differences between these panics and those typical of panic disorders are that they are secondary to some other fear, such as contamination, and are seldom unexpected and inexplicable. The affected person recognizes the connection between the feared situation and the possibility of a panic, and in this important sense, understands the nature of the panic episodes. In contrast, the unexpected, spontaneous panics are bewildering.

People who experience 'situational panics' use their knowledge about their sensitivity to panic in order to develop protective avoidance behaviour. They try to keep away from public lavatories, driving in dense traffic, narrow bridges, frightening movies, or any circumstances that they fear might trigger a panic. They have fewer nasty surprises because they learn to avoid, but at some cost to their ability to move about freely. Situational panics can seriously interfere with a person's life.

What precipitates a panic disorder?

Most panic disorders develop during or after a stressful event or period. Given the unexpected onset of the first few panics, many patients are at a loss to explain their sudden experience of intense fear. However, during assessment and treatment the stressful trigger of the panic tends to emerge.

Major changes in one's life can bring on panics and the most common triggers are: marital/personal conflicts, illness or death of a close person, births or miscarriages, and financial threats or loss, a significant increase in responsibility at home and/or at work. Stress at work, health problems, and negative reactions to drugs are also known to increase the risk of triggering a panic. Disturbing reactions to street drugs can precipitate a panic disorder. The fact that most people endure negative events without panicking, points to the existence of risk factors that make some people especially vulnerable to episodes of panic.

 Case study

Mr T, a successful and busy accountant, was a chronic worrier and easily discouraged. His mother developed a serious incapacitating illness that required him to visit her frequently, and to oversee her health and other needs. His panic episodes began during this period; they were unexpected and extremely frightening. On more than one occasion he felt that he was going to die. Initially, Mr T did not connect the stress of coping with his mother's illness to his panics, which he regarded as an added but independent problem. Later, he described how distressed and over-stretched he had been feeling immediately prior to his first panic. Additionally, his mother's illness had provoked intense fears of his own mortality.

 Case study

Ms C's first episode of panic was precipitated by a bad reaction to smoking cannabis. She began to feel extremely light-headed, out of control, and dizzy, and that her surroundings were unreal. She thought she was going completely insane and was terrified. This initial episode was followed by prolonged anxiety and she became acutely sensitive to unusual tastes or odours. Whenever she felt light-headed or unreal, her anxiety increased and on many occasions she had full panics.

Risk factors

A number of risk factors have been identified: family conflict, separation anxiety during childhood, chronic physical or psychiatric illness in the family, and the abuse of alcohol or drugs in the family. Research on respiratory illnesses indicates that people who have a history of difficulties with their breathing are at increased risk for panic disorder. Panics can be promoted by disturbed personal relationships and/or increases in responsibility.

It has also been found that people who are especially sensitive to their bodily sensations, and are fearful of marked changes in these sensations, are particularly vulnerable to panics. This quality, known as 'anxiety sensitivity', is associated with the frequency and intensity of episodes of fear and panic. People who are anxiety-sensitive worry about the harmful effects of marked changes in their bodily sensations, and endorse questions such as 'I get really scared if my heart starts pounding', ' It scares me when I become short of breath', 'It frightens me whenever I begin to feel faint'. The significance of the bodily sensations is magnified and feeds the person's anxiety. They fear that acute changes might be a sign of a medical or mental disaster, or cause unpleasant social embarrassment (and often believe that other people can easily detect their anxiety). People with elevated anxiety sensitivity are also inclined to anguish over possible harm caused by their repeated episodes of panic.

Elevated anxiety sensitivity is one of a number of predictors of the development of a panic disorder. It is thought of as a vulnerability to panic, but fortunately this excessive sensitivity diminishes during successful psychological treatment.

Genetics

There appears to be a slightly increased risk of panic disorder among people who are born into families in which a close relative has had a diagnosed panic disorder. It is not yet known for certain whether this is because of genetic factors or as a result of their contact with the sufferer. The evidence of panic disorder among sets of identical twins and sets of non-identical twins, which would help to identify a genetic contribution to the disorder, is too sparse to help clear up this point. Genetic factors appear to play a small but significant role in increasing a person's vulnerability to various forms of anxiety disorder, such as obsessive-compulsive disorder. The same may well be true for panic disorder.

Separation anxiety

There is mixed evidence on whether or not separation anxiety in childhood predisposes people to panic disorder in later life. The term 'separation anxiety' refers to the distress exhibited by young children when they are separated, even for brief periods, from a parent, usually the mother. Some people with panic disorder report that they had separation anxiety but the findings, based as they are on the person's recall of childhood events and feelings, may not be reliable. The large majority of children cope well with separations.

The size of the problem

Roughly 15 people out of 1000 in the general population develop a panic disorder at some time in their life. The size of the problem is much the same from country to country, and no ethnic or racial differences have been found. Roughly comparable figures have been reported from different countries, e.g. Canada, Italy, Korea, New Zealand, and the United States.

Persistent panic disorder has an adverse effect on most aspects of the person's life: marital relationship, mobility, social contacts, employment, economic status; it can be extremely disabling. There is a shortage of information about the natural course of (untreated) panic disorder, but the long-term results of a large study of the effects of anti-panic medications provide a rough guide to the outcome of the disorder. Half of the patients showed recurrent or mild symptoms, 30% recovered, and in 20% the panic disorder followed a severe, chronic course. In the most extreme cases the person becomes housebound.

As a group, people who have a panic disorder make greater use of medical services, and the incidence of unemployment or partial employment is higher in this group.

Age and sex

It is relatively rare for the onset of panic disorder to occur before the age of 15, but there are occasional cases in childhood (see p.26). In the majority of cases, the onset occurs in the twenties; in this sense, it is a disorder of early adulthood. While most patients develop their panic disorder for the first time before the age of 40, in rare cases it arises late in life. It is infrequent in people over 65 years old. An example of the development of panic disorder in later life is given in the case study.

 Case study

A 75-year-old woman was tense about travelling to a family reunion at a large, busy hotel and asked her doctor to prescribe a sedative to calm her down for the occasion. She had never before taken this sedative and had an unexpectedly strong reaction to the drug. It made her feel unwell, weak, and increasingly confused, 'until I turned into a zombie'. She remained in a state of distress for two days and was unable to participate in the reunion. Thereafter, whenever she experienced any sensations that were similar to those she had at the hotel (e.g. weakness, palpitations, mental confusion), they induced a panic or near-panic. As a result she feared going out on her own and became almost housebound.

The sex distribution of panic disorders is uneven. In most, but not all, studies there are more female patients than males, mainly because there are more females who have panic disorder with agoraphobia. In this group, the female to male ratio is about 3:1. This may be at least partly due to societal expectations and stereotypes. It has been suggested that females may tend to deal with anticipatory anxiety and fear of panic by avoiding the situations associated with panic attacks, leading to agoraphobia, whereas males may force themselves to confront these situations, not infrequently with the help of alcohol or drugs.

The incidence of alcohol/drug dependence is higher among men with panic disorder than it is in women.

Relation of panic disorder to other disorders

Roughly half of panic disorder patients have been clinically depressed at some time in their lives. Approximately one-quarter have suffered from a social phobia at some time, and the same proportion have had obsessive–compulsive problems. About one in five has abused alcohol and/or drugs.

At the time of diagnosis, many panic disorder patients are also found to have other psychological problems. Roughly 40% have depression concurrent with panic disorder, and it is not clear whether the depressive symptoms in these cases should be seen as an independent disorder, or a result of the restrictions and misery caused by the distress and disablement of the panic disorder. The other disorders commonly associated with panic disorder at diagnosis include social phobia and hypochondriasis. Hypochondriasis is a condition in which the predominant disturbance is extreme anxiety concerning one's health—either the fear that one has a serious illness (e.g. AIDS), or the threat that one is particularly vulnerable to serious illness. (The term hypochondriasis is being replaced with the term 'health anxiety'; either way, there is a common association between this problem and panic disorder.)

A related problem associated with panic disorder is what has been called 'somatization disorder'. This is characterized by recurrent and multiple physical complaints of several years' duration, for which medical help is sought but which are not due to any physical disorder. It generally begins before the age of 30, and has a chronic and fluctuating course. A proportion of these patients have been shown to suffer from panic disorder. In one American study, over half of the patients with somatization disorder were found to satisfy all the diagnostic criteria for panic disorder. As many panic patients tend to complain, under-standably, about their physical symptoms, such as shortness of breath, palpitations, and chest pain, it is likely that the true nature of their disorder is not detected early by doctors in many cases. So they spend many years seeking help for the physical symptoms.

In cases of social phobia, the person has an intense fear of scrutiny and is morbidly self-consciousness. The cognitions dwell on the prospect of a catastrophic social event. In many cases, social phobia and panic disorder are intertwined.

Panic episodes, and frank panic disorder, are commonly found in people with post-traumatic stress disorder (PTSD). Data from people with PTSD arising from road traffic accidents, and those with PTSD caused by exposure to combat stress, have shown that over a quarter have concurrent panic disorder. In these people the panics are sometimes triggered by the intrusive memories or flashbacks of the traumatic event.

Panic in children

A small but significant proportion of adult patients with panic disorder report an onset before the age of 10. Panic disorder is rarely diagnosed in children, but a small number of children and young adolescents do have episodes of panic that are similar to those in adults. The treatment is psychological and the results are satisfactory. In some cases the occurrence of panics is not at first obvious; for example, some children presenting with school phobia or school refusal have been shown to have frequent panic episodes in school settings.

 Case study

Anna was referred for help at the age of 12 because she was generally anxious and was refusing to attend school. During careful assessment, it emerged that Anna had a panic disorder. Her first panic episode occurred at the age of 8 when, in the presence of many other children, she was severely reprimanded by a teacher for being late. She then began to have panics in the school assembly, in the playground when surrounded by other children, and occasionally on her way to school. Anna had several medical examinations before the persistence of her school refusal led to her being referred to a psychological service. She described her panics as involving feelings of weakness, pounding heart, trembling, dizziness, shortness of breath, and a fear that she might die. Most of her panics occurred in or near the school premises, but she also had occasional panics in other places.

The duration of panic disorders

Left untreated, there is a risk that panic disorder can become chronic. In addition, uncontrolled episodes of panic can generate a range of serious other problems, notably agoraphobia. It is depressing to experience these unexpected episodes of intense fear, and to restrict one's life because of them; clinical depression is a common consequence of panic disorder. Some patients attempt to self-medicate, with a range of drugs and/or herbal remedies, and in the most troubling cases, with alcohol. Even though there is a risk that untreated panic disorder can become chronic, a minority of fortunate patients gradually recover without treatment.

Panic disorder and culture

While much of the research on panic disorder has been conducted in Western societies, panic episodes and panic disorder are not limited to this population. Panic disorder has been reported in different cultures and in countries in diverse parts of the world.

The way stress and anxiety are expressed is determined to some extent by one's culture; equally, beliefs about the physical symptoms that one experiences are often culturally determined. These factors sometimes affect the presentation of panic disorder.

Recent research has shown that African Americans tend to report higher levels of physical symptoms in their panic episodes, especially numbing/tingling of extremities, when compared to Caucasian Americans. They also report more intense fears of dying or going crazy. Hispanic Americans are reported to show a culture-specific reaction termed '*ataque de nervios*'. Typically, this occurs during severe stress. Many of the symptoms are the same as those of panic disorder and, indeed, it has been reported that the majority of Hispanic patients who have '*ataque de nervios*' and panic disorder use the term '*ataque*' to describe their panic episodes.

Among the Chinese, dizziness is a common symptom of distress. This is seen as reflecting disharmony/disequilibrium. Patients with panic disorder, or those with symptoms that would warrant a diagnosis of panic disorder, are said to have dizziness as a prominent symptom.

There is also some interesting information about panic in Cambodian people. In a study of Khmer refugee patients in the United States, a type of panic disorder was identified that has been called 'the sore neck syndrome'. In these patients, the most commonly reported fear was that of dying as the result of a rupture in a neck vessel, caused by high blood and wind pressure.

The experience of panic and the manifestations of panic disorder transcend cultural and ethnic boundaries.

4

The consequences of panic

→ Key Points

- The main consequences of panic are a build-up of anxious apprehension and the development of pervasive patterns of avoidance.

- The fear of experiencing another panic can have major effects on the person's appraisal of danger and safety.

- Given the fear of further panics, the person's pattern of avoidance has a logic of its own.

- The underlying catastrophic thoughts determine which places/situations are potentially dangerous and best avoided.

- The most commonly avoided places/situations are described; they include driving, travelling alone, shopping, social occasions, public transport.

- In severe cases, the fear and avoidance prevent the person from working, taking part in social activities, establishing/maintaining personal relationships.

- Sufferers from the disorder tend to over-predict when and where they are likely to panic.

- During treatment and/or self-directed exposure exercises the predictions gradually become more accurate.

- The expectations of panic are mainly stable but odd fluctuations do occur; for example, many sufferers report that on occasions they can tell on awakening whether or not they are likely to panic during the day.

Most episodes of panic are distressing, but the psychological consequences can be disabling and persist for years. As described in Chapter 3, after a number of panic episodes, it is likely that the affected person will begin to avoid particular places and activities. The avoidance can become so severe as to shape and limit their entire life—personal life, marriage, employment, social life, recreation. In extreme cases the person is unable to leave the house except when accompanied, and then only for short distances and brief periods. For these people the impact of the disorder can leave them virtually disabled. Unemployment or partial employment rates are elevated among people who have the disorder; they make greater use of medical services than do other people.

The pattern of the avoidance behaviour is determined by the person's particular fears. Someone who fears that exertion might bring on a heart attack will avoid energetic actions such as sports. A person who fears that he/she may lose control and jump off a high place will avoid bridges and tall buildings. A person who fears AIDS will avoid hospitals, rundown areas, public lavatories, and if he inadvertently or unavoidably touches a contaminant, may well panic. A person who fears suffocation will avoid tunnels, elevators, tube trains, and may be prone to panic if he feels trapped in one of these situations. The activities and situations that are most commonly avoided are driving, travelling alone, shopping, social occasions, public transport.

The main concern behind this avoidance behaviour is to ensure one's safety, and to have easy and rapid access to safety in all potentially risky situations. For example, the person may avoid being alone at home in case of a medical disaster, or travelling alone, or ensure that a car is always available and reliable, that they always sit on the aisle and near an exit, and avoid shopping unaccompanied, avoid waiting in queues, or ensure that the hotel room is on the ground level and is well-aired.

A list of common forms of avoidance is provided from the Mobility Inventory (Table 4.1) developed by Dr Diane Chambless and her colleagues. The Inventory is reproduced in Appendix 1.

Episodes of panic usually engender feelings of anxious apprehension. It is common to feel anxious for periods each day, accompanied by feelings of restlessness and irritability. Worry, preoccupation with the panics and their significance, and feelings of depression are common consequences of panic episodes.

As described in Chapter 1, there is a common transition from the fear of a medical or physical disaster to a fear of having another episode of panic. There is a close connection between the person's fear of another panic and particular forms of avoidance. They will strictly avoid any and all situations in which they anticipate that a panic is likely to occur. One patient said, 'I keep away from the market because I know a panic is certain to occur'. Other examples are: 'I avoid using elevators because I *know* that I will panic'; 'I dare not travel on a bus or train because I will panic'; 'It is useless looking for work because I am not capable of turning up regularly'.

In general, the person's expectation of a panic is the strongest determinant of avoidance on a particular day in a particular place. If they predict that a panic is highly likely, the place or event will be avoided. However, if they anticipate that no panic or other disaster will occur in that particular place at that time, then there is no need or urge to avoid.

Table 4.1 Common forms of avoidance

Going in airplanes
Being far away from home
Underground and tunnels
Going in ships/boats
Theatres
Going in buses
Going in trains
Museums
Stadiums/auditoriums
High places
Driving on motorways
Department stores
Restaurants
Enclosed places
Standing in queues
Parties
Crossing bridges
Supermarkets

From Chambless *et al.* (1985). See Appendix 5 for full reference. Reproduced with permission.

Most sufferers from panic disorder experience fluctuations in their anxiety and their expectations of panic. They have good days and bad days and sometimes know on waking what to expect. In part these fluctuations are caused by changes in mood but it is also possible to make sense of many fluctuations by close analysis of the person's thoughts about the possibility of disaster.

The mere fact that the anxiety, expectations of panic, and especially the avoidance behaviour do fluctuate, can be a source of misunderstanding and conflict within the family. It is commonly believed that a person's behaviour is, or should be, consistent from day to day. And the ability to travel to work unaccompanied, to take one example, should be consistent. An irate relative who says: 'Why must I travel with you today when you were perfectly capable of going on your own yesterday?' reflects the belief that people should be consistent in their behaviour. To the observer, especially close family members or friends, the variability in the sufferer's avoidance behaviour, and in the demands made upon friends and relatives, is puzzling. The reasons for these fluctuations are seldom obvious, even to the sufferer, and add to the irrational quality of panic disorders. The variability sometimes calls into question the authenticity of the sufferer's

problem: Are they genuinely panicky? Do they really need me to stay at home with them? Is there perhaps an element of exaggeration or pretending? Sometimes the inexplicable fluctuations in the patient's anxiety/avoidance are mistakenly interpreted as a sign of deep mental instability.

The fear of panicking does have irrational qualities, just as many other fears have an irrational element, such as intense fears of harmless spiders. It is important to recognize that a person who experiences apparently irrational panics is not wholly irrational or mentally unstable. There are irrational features in almost all forms of human behaviour; we all think and behave irrationally at times without being considered psychologically abnormal.

After a few episodes of panic, people begin to make informal predictions about if and when they will experience another panic. After an unexpected panic they are likely to think that the next panic is far more probable than it really is. As mentioned earlier, such over-prediction is very common. Far more episodes of panic are expected than ever occur.

The tendency to expect the worst is, however, modifiable. With repeated experiences of panics, and of periods/places free of panic, the sufferer's predictions become more accurate, and they learn to anticipate reasonably well when and where panics are likely to occur. Just as the predictions of further panics are modifiable, so predictions of a safe period are also modifiable, although it takes many more experiences of safety to reassure the sufferer that a panic is very unlikely to occur. Fear and anxiety are quickly increased by a panic episode, but regaining confidence about one's safety is a considerably slower process. The process can be facilitated by systematic treatment—the frequency and intensity of episodes of panic diminish and the undesirable consequences fade out.

5

Theories of panic disorder

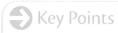 Key Points

- There are two approaches to understanding the causes of panic disorders.

- The first approach, introduced by Klein, established the nature and distinctiveness of panic disorders.

- His original explanation was replaced by the idea that everyone has an in-born suffocation-alarm system, and that those people who possess a super-sensitive alarm system are vulnerable to panics.

- It is a biological explanation and the suggested treatment is a course of medication.

- The second approach is psychological and proposes that panics occur when the person makes a catastrophic misinterpretation of certain bodily sensations, such as a pounding heart or difficulty breathing, or makes a catastrophic interpretation of benign events.

- The suggested treatment is cognitive-behaviour therapy, in which attempts are made to assist the patient make more realistic and adaptive interpretations of sensations and/or events. The therapy includes changes in behaviour with an emphasis on reducing the person's unadaptive avoidance.

- The effectiveness of both forms of treatment is supported by credible evidence.

- Numbers of patients receive a combination of psychological therapy and medication.

There are two main approaches to understanding the cause of panic disorders: one that emphasizes biological factors and the other that emphasizes psychological factors. It is widely agreed that both biological and psychological factors are involved, but opinions differ on the relative importance of each type, and how they combine. At present there is no fully satisfactory and comprehensive explanation of panic disorder, but progress has been made. As with some other medical and psychological problems, the absence of a full explanation of panic disorder has not precluded the development of effective treatment methods. Therapeutic progress often precedes theoretical explanations.

The biological theory

The occurrence of episodes of panic is not new, but in the 1960s a psychiatrist at the New York Psychiatric Institute, Dr Donald Klein, suggested that people who repeatedly experience severe panics, especially unexpected panics, are suffering from a separate and distinctive disorder: panic disorder. After a good deal of research, his suggestion was accepted, and in 1980 the diagnosis of panic disorder was included in the major classification system of the American Psychiatric Association. The classifications are set out in the Association's *Diagnostic and Statistical Manual*, the DSM, which has been adopted in many countries. Dr Klein based his proposal on two main pieces of evidence. First, he observed that patients who experienced severe, unexpected panics failed to respond to medications that reduced most other types of anxiety disorder, but surprisingly did respond favourably to one drug, imipramine (see p.41), which is used mainly as a treatment for depression. He concluded, therefore, that the panic sufferers were different from the patients who had other forms of anxiety disorder.

Secondly, in laboratory research, many of the panic sufferers experienced attacks when sodium lactate was infused into them. Fewer patients with other types of anxiety disorder responded in this way to this lactate test, and Dr Klein used these results to strengthen his suggestion that repeated episodes of panic indicate the presence of a separate and distinctive disorder. Moreover, when panic patients were medicated with the anti-depressant drug imipramine, they were far less likely to panic during the lactate test. Dr Klein concluded that that the drug blocked the laboratory panics, and hence supported a biological explanation of panic disorders.

He proposed that panic disorders are primarily biological in nature: patients have a super-sensitive alarm system that is repeatedly and unexpectedly triggered by pathological discharges in the nervous system, causing spontaneous panics. These discharges are thought to be linked to fears of suffocation, or separation anxiety. The spontaneous panics occur at unpredictable times, including nocturnal panics, and can occur in unexpected places. The experience of spontaneous panics gives rise to apprehension about further episodes, increased anxiety, and eventually agoraphobia.

Dr Klein's work was extremely influential and his main suggestion, that panic disorder is a separate disorder, is accepted. In addition, the link between panic and subsequent fear and avoidance has been confirmed.

The theory of a pathological central discharge in the nervous system has fared less well, and indeed Dr Klein has revised his original ideas. The problems began when it was found that, contrary to the initial reports, patients with panic disorder did in fact respond favourably to certain drugs that are effective in treating other forms of anxiety disorder. Panic disorders do not respond only and distinctively to a particular, anti-depressant drug. (See Chapter 6 for the range of current medications.)

The second plank in Dr Klein's theory, that panic disorder patients respond distinctively and predictably to the sodium lactate laboratory test, was not confirmed. Later research revealed that patients with disorders other than panic disorder, and even some people free of any disorder, can also give similar responses to the test. Furthermore, the original idea, that most panic disorder patients have attacks when given sodium lactate, had to be revised; the revised estimates were that roughly 50% of panic disorder patients give this response, rather than the 85% originally thought to do so. As it was originally believed that the laboratory test is effective because it triggered a central discharge of the over-sensitive alarm system, the growing numbers of different responses among panic disorder patients presented a problem. It meant that even if the theory is correct, it might apply only to a subset of panic disorder patients. Moreover, the fact that numbers of non-panic disorder patients also gave similar responses to the test had not been predicted.

It was also pointed out that the distinction between the spontaneous panics, to which Dr Klein attached great importance, and the other more common panics, is not as clear as implied in the theory. Critics also complained that the theory was vague on significant details.

In a revision of the theory, Dr Klein suggested that we are all equipped with a sensitive, in-born suffocation alarm system. However, if that system is too easily and/or too frequently set off, it can cause 'spontaneous' panics. It follows that the underlying problem for many, or most, panic disorder sufferers is a super-sensitive suffocation alarm system. It certainly is the case that many sufferers of panic disorder experience breathing difficulties and that an intense fear of suffocation can be an important factor among these people.

The suffocation alarm theory is plausible but research has not confirmed its validity. Even if the suffocation alarm theory is not the key, it has led to a useful distinction between emergency reactions to a genuine threat (a true alarm) and emergency reactions to false alarms. In Klein's theory, the false alarms arise from a firing of the over-sensitive suffocation alarm system in non-threatening circumstances. The division into true alarms and false alarms is also central to the psychological explanation of panics.

Dr Klein's account is only one of several biological theories of panic disorder. Theorists have put forward different views of a biological cause, with some suggestive evidence. Overall, none of these is conclusively supported at present.

Psychological theories

The observation of breathing difficulties in panic disorder patients sparked off what later became the most influential alternative to Dr Klein's biological theory.

Like many clinicians before and since, Professor David Clark, of the Institute of Psychiatry at King's College, University of London, noted the frequency with which these patients experience breathing difficulties. Their breathing tends to be too rapid and/or too shallow. The effects of over-breathing (hyperventilation) often include dizziness, feeling light-headed, rapid heart beat, unsteadiness, tingling of the extremities, tightness of the chest, and even a sense of unreality.

Among panic disorder sufferers, episodes of panic can be precipitated by over-breathing. Dr Clark's observations led him to believe that the panics occur when the person thinks that the effects of over-breathing (such as light-headedness, feelings of unreality, chest pressure) mean that something terrible is about to happen. For example: 'My chest is tight and I feel dizzy and faint, which means I am having a heart attack. I am about to die'. Dr Clark expanded his work beyond the study of over-breathing to include a range of unpleasant and/or unexplained bodily sensations and then introduced a fresh explanation for panic disorder.

People become extremely frightened when they feel that they are in immediate danger, and react accordingly. Their emergency reactions consist of intense physical sensations, such as a pounding heart, difficulty breathing, and catastrophic thoughts. If, however, there is no real danger, if it is a false alarm, the emergency reactions are distressing and unadaptive. Dr Clark proposed that episodes of panic are caused by a serious misinterpretation of various bodily sensations or thoughts—they are false alarms.

The most common misinterpretations that provoke a panic are: a fear of an imminent heart attack, a fear of suffocation, a fear of completely losing control, a fear of going insane, a fear of choking, a fear of public embarrassment/humiliation, a fear of a brain tumour or other serious disease. People who are predisposed to fear one or more of these personal catastrophes, either because of their personal or family history, and who are acutely sensitive to their bodily sensations, are at increased risk of developing panic disorder.

Any event or situation that provokes unpleasant bodily sensations, such as faintness caused by over-breathing, is open to misinterpretation. A person who is especially frightened of an early death by a sudden heart attack, say because of a family history of heart trouble, may misinterpret tightness in his/her chest when exercising as a symptom of a coming attack, and panic. However, if that same person explains the feeling as a normal response to exercising, then he/she will not panic.

Where do these catastrophic thoughts come from? In most cases the thoughts are traceable to the sufferer's personal experiences (for example, a history of breathing problems such as asthma, or a life-threatening episode of choking) or to serious illnesses, death, or catastrophes that they have witnessed, or heard about, in close relatives or friends. For example, the patient described on p.67

was frightened of developing a fatal recurrence of cancer just as her mother and aunt had done. Another patient feared that his occasional feelings of 'unreality' were a sign that he would become schizophrenic and be confined in a long-stay hospital, as had the uncle whom he visited in a psychiatric hospital. These visits, which began when the patient was an adolescent, were always distressing and he was anxiously aware of thinking that he might follow his uncle into insanity. Another example comes from a man of 45 who had been troubled by anxiety about his health for many years, despite repeated reassurances from physicians. One fine day he had a sudden episode of intense fear while starting to play a round of golf. His heart was pounding and he had such difficulty breathing that he thought he was having a heart attack and asked his companions to call for an ambulance. At the hospital emergency room he was reassured and advised to consult a psychologist or psychiatrist. It turned out that 3 months earlier a close family friend had experienced a major heart attack on the golf course and died a few days later. Without realizing it at the time, the patient had been ruminating about the sudden death of his friend as he approached the golf course and felt unwell and anxious. When his heart started pounding he was terrified that he too was having a heart attack. This case illustrates how negative information coming from indirect or direct sources can prime catastrophic thoughts, and they can be elicited when the person experiences unpleasant bodily sensations and/or enters a situation that is associated with threat and fears. Misfortunes or catastrophes that have occurred to family or friends are a common and powerful source of negative expectations; they prime the vulnerable person's store of disturbing memories. Intrusive, recurrent images of disturbing memories are remarkably vivid, emotionally-charged and unchanging. Some images are traceable to events in adolescence or childhood, and themes of abandonment, being trapped, suffocating, are common.

These fearful, negative memories and recurrent, intrusive images of catastrophic events can be extraordinarily persistent and haunt the person for many, many years.

To summarize: the perception of unpleasant/unexplained bodily sensations and/or catastrophic thoughts/images, can cause a panic reaction. If the person makes a catastrophic misinterpretation of the sensations and/or the negative thoughts, a panic is likely to follow. If the person makes a safe, benign interpretation of the sensations or images, there will be no panic.

Case study

A 25-year-old woman, with no history of psychological troubles, was voluntarily taking part in a laboratory demonstration of the effects of standing in a small, enclosed space (a sort of telephone kiosk in this particular experiment) for up to two minutes. To her surprise she had felt hot and flushed in the enclosed space and began to sweat profusely. Her breathing was rapid and shallow, she became acutely upset by a feeling of being trapped, and then panicked. Later, she explained that she had thought she was about to faint and completely lose control of herself.

When asked if she had ever experienced similar physical sensations (flushes, sweating, shortness of breath) at other times, she promptly replied that it reminded her of how she felt after jogging. She then added, 'But that has never bothered me because I know that exercise causes sweating and panting'. A benign interpretation of the same physical sensations produced no fear.

Clark and his colleagues were able to show that panic disorder patients not only report lots of spontaneously occurring frightening thoughts, but that if the patients are encouraged to produce the relevant physical sensations (such as over-breathing) and also make a worrying interpretation of the sensations, intense fear can be evoked. Panic disorder patients are also vulnerable to situational panics. Situations or activities that they associate with danger (such as a danger of contracting serious contamination), or memories of danger, can evoke panics.

A simple diagram illustrating the cognitive model of panic is given in Figure 5.1. In Figure 5.2, a specific example of a patient's panic attack is provided.

Dr Clark's psychological theory, and a similar theory developed independently by Dr David Barlow of Boston University, can account for many aspects of panic disorder, including the previously puzzling fact that some patients experience panics when they begin to feel deeply relaxed. These so-called relaxation panics occur among people who fear if they lose control then a catastrophe, such as death or an insane action, will occur. They feel they must hold on to their conscious control in all of their waking hours, or else …. These fears sometimes have their origin in disturbing experiences with illegal drugs. Negative reactions to these drugs frequently produce disturbances of vision/sound, feelings of unreality, and a terrifying loss of control. Not surprisingly, people who have endured these frightening reactions are resistant to taking any drugs, even prescribed ones.

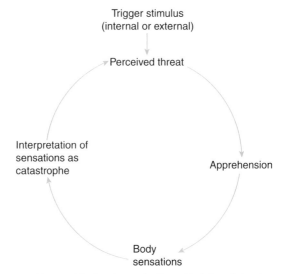

Figure 5.1 A cognitive model of panic attacks. From Clark (1986). See Appendix 5 for full reference. Reproduced with permission.

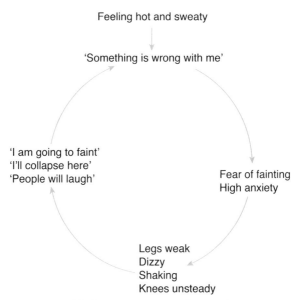

Figure 5.2 Cognitive model of panic attacks: a specific example.

The psychological theories have their limitations, and cannot explain fully the occurrence of nocturnal panics, and of some of the effects of therapy. As will be described in Chapter 6, the therapy that grew out of the psychological approach is effective, but some forms of psychological therapy, which pay little attention to the patient's interpretations of their sensations and thoughts, are also effective. The question that then arises is whether the change from misinterpretations to correct interpretations is indeed a necessary part of effective treatment. If some patients improve even without any deliberate attempt to correct the misinterpretations, then it follows such corrections of misinterpretations can take place spontaneously, or may not be essential for producing improvements.

The general reasoning about panic, in which catastrophic cognitions are central, is also applicable to the related disorders of social phobia and health anxiety. The primary difference between a panic disorder and an intense, extreme anxiety about one's health, is that in panics, the person feels in imminent danger, but in health anxiety, the fear is of a catastrophic illness occurring at some time in the future, e.g. developing cancer.

From theory to treatment

Both the biological and psychological theories have been used as a foundation for the development of treatments for panic disorder. The biological approach has spawned a continuous search for effective new drugs, especially those with minimal side-effects. The psychological approach gave rise to cognitive-behavioural therapy, in which patients are guided towards more appropriate interpretations of their experiences, and are taught how to reduce the intensity and frequency of their disturbing bodily sensations. These are discussed in Chapters 6 and 7.

For readers who wish to consider detailed accounts of the theories, and critical commentaries on them, some of the key references are given in the annotated reading list provided in Appendix 5.

6

Treatment of panic disorder

Key Points

- Panic disorder is treatable.
- Cognitive behaviour therapy consists of detailed analyses of the exact nature of the patient's fears, and the basis on which they rest.
- These analyses are combined with exercises designed primarily to reduce the unadaptive avoidance behaviour.
- A course of this psychological treatment usually takes between 8 and 12 sessions, and is provided by a clinical psychologist.
- Group treatment of panic disorder is reasonably effective.
- Three classes of medication are available for the treatment of the disorder.
- Medications are prescribed by medical practitioners, and are selected to meet the particular needs of the individual patient.
- The medications have a slow build-up and it takes from 2 to 8 weeks for the full effects to be felt.
- Most of the medications are accompanied by some side-effects, and termination of the medication must be tapered in order to avoid negative discontinuation effects.

Panic disorder is a treatable disorder. In 2004 the National Institute of Health and Clinical Excellence (NICE) published a comprehensive review of the evidence pertaining to the treatment of panic disorder and/or agoraphobia, and made explicit recommendations. There are two effective forms of treatment: psychological therapy (notably cognitive behaviour therapy) and medication. The panel of experts who participated in a consensus conference on panic disorder organized by the National Institutes of Health of the United States, reached the same conclusions. Psychological treatments are of 'demonstrated efficacy in the reduction and/or elimination of panic attacks and agoraphobia … significant numbers of patients are panic-free at the end of … treatment and remain so at a two-year follow-up'. The treatment is well-tolerated and acceptable to most patients. In addition, certain classes of medication 'have been found to be effective in reducing or eliminating panic attacks associated with the various forms of panic disorder' (Wolfe and Maser 1994).

An abridged version of the NICE report is available at: www.nice.org.uk/CG022quickrefguide

Medication

Medication is widely used for treating panic disorder. As originally reported by Dr D.Klein, the tricyclic anti-depressant drug imipramine (Tofranil®) is a demonstrably effective treatment for panic disorder. Imipramine generally blocks the episodes of panic and reduces the patient's general anxiety. Depression, as noted in an earlier chapter, is a common accompaniment of panic disorder and imipramine can serve a double purpose by reducing panic disorder and depression. All of these medications require a prescription from a medical doctor. Psychologists provide psychological treatment but do not prescribe medications.

The drug is usually given in small doses initially, e.g. 25 mg, and gradually increased by 25 mg every three days to an average 150 mg per day, over a period of two to three weeks. Many patients require high doses for the drug to be effective, in some cases as high as 300 mg per day. The beneficial effects of the medication tend to appear roughly two to four weeks after treatment begins. The possible side-effects include: dry mouth, blurred vision, nausea, light-headedness, urinary retention, constipation, weight gain, over-stimulation, drowsiness, postural-hypotension, sweating, and sexual difficulties. In many cases patients become accustomed to the drug and the side-effects diminish. However, between one-quarter and one-third of patients experience side-effects that lead them to discontinue the medication. Before starting the medication patients are prepared by the provision of full information and an explanation of the therapeutic benefits and the expected side-effects. They are informed that the effects of the medication take a few weeks to become apparent, and they are advised not to stop taking the medication abruptly as they might experience adverse 'discontinuation' effects for several days or longer. These medications are not habit-forming and do not produce drug dependence.

Patients tend to be kept on the medication for up to 12 months. The drug is tapered off gradually and carefully, usually over a period of two to three months, in order to avoid negative reactions. Unfortunately, when the medications are finally discontinued there is a possibility of relapse. The drug should not be taken by people who have cardiac disorders, mania, urinary difficulties, and glaucoma. Imipramine should never be taken at the same time as other anti-depressants, particularly those in MAOI group (see below). Other tricyclic anti-depressants that have anti-panic effects include clomipramine (Anafranil®) and nortriptyline (Allegron®).

A second type of anti-depressant medication, the monoamine oxidase inhibitors (MAOI), has also been shown to be effective, but is less frequently prescribed because of side-effects, adverse interactions with other medications, and the need to adopt a restrictive diet. The possible side-effects include: dry mouth, constipation, blurred vision, postural hypotension, insomnia, sexual problems, and weight gain. It is not suitable for people with blood pressure problems, cardiovascular disorders or headaches, and should not be taken at the same time as other anti-depressants, or with any of a range of other medications. Foods or preparations that contain tyramine (including cheese, beer, red wine and meat extracts) are prohibited. The list of precautions for MAOI drugs is lengthy and care must be taken with these prescriptions. The medication is introduced slowly after giving the patient a full explanation of the benefits, risks, and dietary/medication restrictions. The starting dose is usually 15 mg daily, and this is slowly increased to 45–60 mg a day, and in some cases up to 90 mg a day. The exact amounts vary slightly from one type of MAOI to the next, and detailed instructions are necessary with each. A commonly used drug of this class in the treatment of panic disorder is phenelzine (Nardil®). Another MAOI that is used is tranyl-cypromine (Parnate®). Isocarboxazid (Marplan® was the former brand name for this) is also used.

Common foods and drinks that should be avoided by patients on MAOI drugs are listed in Table 6.1.

Table 6.1 Dietary restrictions for patients taking MAOI drugs

Common foods to be avoided
Beer
Broad bean pods
Cheese*
Dry sausage
Foods containing cheese (such as pizza)
Liver
Meat extracts
Over-ripe bananas
Red wine
Smoked or pickled fish, especially herring
Sour cream
Yeast extracts
Yogurt

*Except cottage cheese and cream cheese in moderate quantities.

Note: This is not an exhaustive list.

Some members of a class of drugs that are known to reduce anxiety, the benzo-diazepines, can reduce panic frequency but are no longer recommended by NICE because the results are less good than those produced by other types of medication. The drug alprazolam (Xanax®), a high-potency benzodiazepine, has been widely prescribed for panic disorder. However, withdrawal can be difficult with benzodiazepines, and it is therefore desirable to taper off the dosage slowly. The relapse rate after terminating the medication is high; in some reports up to 90%.

The common side-effects include sleeplessness, light-headedness, and slowing of physical and mental activity. Less common effects include fatigue, slurred speech, and forgetfulness. There are risks of dependence with benzodiazepines, and for this reason they are not prescribed for patients who have a history of alcohol or drug abuse. The exact dose varies between medications, but alprazolam is generally started at a low dose of 0.5 mg, three times daily, increasing up to 6 mg daily. In some cases a dose of 10 mg is needed. The increase in the dosage is done in small steps, and abrupt withdrawal of the medication is avoided. Two other benzodiazepines, clonazepam (Rivotril®) and lorazepam (Ativan®), have also been used in the treatment of panic disorder. As noted, benzodiazepines are less effective overall than other medications.

In recent years, anti-depressants of the SSRI (selective serotonin re-uptake inhibitors) group have been used with success. The drugs used include fluoxetine (Prozac®), fluvoxamine (Faverin®), sertraline (Lustral®), citalopram (Cipramil®) and paroxetine (Seroxat®). These tend to have fewer side-effects than the tricyclics. However, some patients may develop problems such as restlessness, agitation, and insomnia, and for this reason the treatment is started with relatively small dosages gradually building up. The drop-out rate tends to be lower for SSRI drugs than for other anti-depressants.

In summary, imipramine is still widely used for panic disorder. If imipramine is poorly tolerated or insufficient, other anti-depressants from the same group are used. The MAOI anti-depressants offer another possibility, and are used with particular care because of the risks and prohibitions. The use of SSRI anti-depressants has increased because the positive evidence has accumulated, and because the side-effects appear to be better tolerated than those of other drugs. Many clinicians now consider SSRI drugs to be the first-choice medication for panic disorder.

As mentioned, benzodiazepines are no longer recommended by NICE, and anti-psychotic medications are definitely discouraged.

The decision about what medication to use and at what dosage, depends on the doctor's assessment and the patient's experiences with drugs and preferences. There are individual differences in reaction to the various drugs and often it is necessary to go through a period of trial and error before finding the medication that is most effective and most tolerable for the particular patient.

During prolonged treatment, shifts between drugs are common. The patient is prescribed different medications at different times—and, not uncommonly, at the same time. However, the effects of simultaneous multiple prescriptions can be confusing and difficult to evaluate. Some patients are reluctant to take medication because the side-effects are not tolerable and/or they have reservations about taking psychiatric drugs. In treatment research trials, a significant minority of participants decline to take drugs, or take them for a period and then withdraw from the research because of the side-effects.

The possible side-effects of the medications, which differ for each particular drug, can be an obstacle and the development of more easily tolerated medications would be very welcome. The list of side-effects for the various drugs can include nausea, dry mouth, headaches, dizziness, weight gain, sexual difficulties, urinary retention, constipation, sweating, sleepiness. Detailed information about the drugs that can be used for panic disorders is readily available on authoritative web-sites.

Psychological treatment

Prior to the recognition of panic disorder as a distinct condition, most people who suffered from panics,and who also feared and avoided public places, buses, trains, markets, enclosed places, and driving, were given the diagnosis of agoraphobia. Up until the seventies, the focus was on agoraphobia and the occurrence of episodes of panic was regarded as an incidental feature of agoraphobia. Hence the first psychological treatment was developed for the management of agoraphobia.

The main psychological treatment for agoraphobia was systematic desensitization to the feared places, and/or planned exercises that consisted of entering the feared places for increasingly long periods. With both of these techniques, the affected person is gradually and systematically exposed to the objects of their fears: in the classical version, systematic desensitization, the exposures take place in imagined rehearsals during relaxation; and in the second treatment, the exposures take place in the real situations. Both methods are examples of 'behaviour therapy'. In most cases nowadays the exposure treatment is carried out in the real situations because the evidence from research trials consistently showed that it was superior to imaginary exposures. Planned, repeated and graded exposures to the feared situations are the mainstay of current treatment for agoraphobia.

Over the years the results of research produced a shift in emphasis from agoraphobia to panic disorders, as it became evident that episodes of panic often are the underlying problem, the cause of the agoraphobia. This advance in understanding contributed to the introduction of an important new component to the prevailing behavioural treatment. Therapists began to focus their attention on eliciting the patient's cognitions about their fears and panics—their thoughts, beliefs, ideas pertaining to the fears, and the thoughts they experience during the panics. With this information, attempts are made to modify those cognitions that are unadaptive, erroneous, harmful. This expansion of behaviour therapy is appropriately labelled cognitive-behaviour therapy—a combination of cognitive and behavioural techniques. In most cases the initial part of the treatment focuses on the patient's cognitions, and the behavioural elements are added after three or four sessions. This method is the best established psychological treatment for panic disorder. Before describing the details of the treatment, some background information may be helpful.

Behaviour therapy, also called behaviour modification or behavioural psycho-therapy, refers to the use of learning theory in the treatment of psychological disorders. Learning theory is the body of knowledge and ideas that psychologists have developed on the basis of hundreds of studies of how changes take place in human and animal behaviour. The use of this knowledge for managing psychological disorders was considered a possibility, and several people took up the challenge. When sufficient progress had been made, rudimentary treatment techniques were introduced in the 1950s. Dr Joseph Wolpe (1916–97), a South African psychiatrist who later practised in Temple University, Philadelphia, pioneered one of the most successful methods. The work of Hans Eysenck at the Institute in London contributed greatly to the development and acceptance of behaviour therapy as a major approach to certain psychological problems. Many behaviour problems are viewed as learned behaviour, as cases of faulty or 'maladaptive' learning, or as cases of failure to learn. The aim was to correct the disorder by applying the principles of learning: the faulty learning can be undone and new learning can be promoted. Therefore, behaviour therapy concentrates on the problem behaviour itself, rather than an assumed root cause. This is in contrast to the psychoanalytic approach of Sigmund Freud (1856–1937) and his followers who regarded the behavioural problems as symptoms of a deeper, unconscious problem. Behaviour therapists concentrate on the problem as it is now, and the factors that are maintaining it. Therapists need to know from the patient when the problem started, how it developed, and so on, but the main focus is on the problem as it is now and the therapist's efforts are geared towards modifying the maladaptive thoughts and behaviour.

The efficacy of behaviour therapy for a range of psychological disorders is well-established. For many of these, it is now considered by many clinicians to be the treatment of choice. An early criticism of this method was that if the problem is treated directly by behaviour therapy without going into its presumed unconscious roots, new symptoms will emerge. This concern was ultimately shown to be unfounded.

Cognitive-behaviour therapy is the result of expanding the scope of behaviour therapy to include aspects of what is known as cognitive therapy, which focuses the patient's cognitions. The most impressive early work by cognitive therapists was in the treatment of depression. Depressed patients usually suffer from negative thoughts such as: 'I am a worthless person', 'There is no future for me',

'There is no point in my life', and so on. Attempts are made to modify these using a variety of techniques, including challenging the maladaptive thoughts, showing evidence to the contrary, and setting up situations in which they are disconfirmed.

The value of cognitive-behaviour therapy was first established in managing depression, and the principles and techniques were then adapted for treating anxiety disorders such as panic disorder.

Cognitive behaviour therapy (CBT)

Exposure exercises

The exercises that were developed for the treatment of agoraphobia retain their value in the treatment of panic disorder, particularly if the patient's activities and travel have become restricted. In the original exposure method (systematic desensitization), the patient was given a course of relaxation training and then asked to imagine the fearful situations/activities while in a state of deep relaxation. The fearful images are ranked from least to most disturbing and presented in a graded and gradual manner starting with least fearful. The ranking is commonly done on the basis of the subjective fear ratings given by the patient, usually on a 0–100 scale (see p.72). With repeated practice the images become less and less fearful, and the patient is then urged to facilitate the transfer of these increasingly fearless reactions from imagination into the real situation.

For example, while relaxing, the patient who is afraid of travelling by bus might start by imagining riding in a bus for one stop. After several repetitions, the fear reaction will decline. After overcoming an item in the list, the patient then tackles the next most fearful item. When the patient's fears have reduced and they are ready, they will be encouraged to actually take a short bus ride. The whole process is gradual, methodical, and progressive—and cushioned by relaxation.

Unfortunately, systematic desensitization can be a lengthy process, and the transfer from fearless imagination to fearless performance is by no means assured. In many instances the transfer is incomplete or simply fails to occur.

For reasons of efficiency and superior therapeutic results, the imaginal exposure technique was largely replaced by exposure exercises that take place in the real situations, so-called *in vivo* exposure. As with systematic desensitization, a list of fearful situations is compiled, ranging from the least to the most frightening, which is then used in planning the exposure exercises, which take place daily, if possible, or as frequently as is practical. The hierarchy is used flexibly, depending on the circumstances, but the plan is to move progressively from the least to the most frightening situation.

The following is a simplified example of a fear hierarchy:

1. walking to the gate of a nearby park, accompanied by a trusted adult;
2. walking 100 yards into the park, accompanied;

3. staying in the park for 10 minutes, accompanied;
4. walking to the gate of the park, alone;
5. walking into the park, alone.

The patient is required to keep a diary that includes each exercise and the degree of anxiety present before, during, and after the exercise, plus the time and distances, and any panicky feelings. An example of a record sheet from such a diary is given in Figure 8.2.

To continue the example:

Item 1, walking to nearby park, accompanied, 30 minutes, April 12, a.m.
    Anxiety before = 80/100
    Anxiety during = 70/100
    Anxiety after = 55/100
Item 1, repeat, 30 minutes, April 13, a.m.
    Anxiety before = 60/100
    Anxiety during = 50/100
    Anxiety after = 30/100
Item 2, walking 100 yards into park, accompanied, 45 minutes, April 14, a.m.
    Anxiety before = 65/100
    Anxiety during = 30/100
    Anxiety after = 20/100

In most instances the first few exposure exercises are carried out while accompanied by a therapist or aide. As the patient's fear begins to subside with repeated exercises, the therapist gradually distances him/herself in a planned manner, and finally fades out of the picture altogether.

As in systematic desensitization, relaxation can be used as a technique for suppressing fear. Typically, patients are trained to relax themselves, and then encouraged to induce feelings of relaxation before and during exposure exercises, and whenever they begin to feel high levels of anxiety.

Cognitive therapy of panic

Cognitive therapy is based on the idea that panics are caused by catastrophic misinterpretations of certain bodily sensations (see Chapter 5). Therefore, in order to eliminate panics, it is necessary to modify the catastrophic misinterpretations and encourage the formation of more accurate and realistic appraisals. Additionally attempts are made to reduce the severity and frequency with which the person experiences the bodily sensations. This has several benefits. The introduction or restoration of safer and more realistic interpretations of these sensations should ensure that few, or no, panics are experienced.

Furthermore, a reduction in the severity and frequency of the bodily sensations will reduce the likelihood of making catastrophic misinterpretations. Finally, therapy usually includes steps to combat any maladaptive avoidance behaviour that has emerged as a consequence of the episodes of panic.

Identification

In order to modify the maladaptive cognitions it is necessary first to identify them. After obtaining a full description of the type and frequency of panic episodes that the person has experienced, the next step is to obtain a detailed description of a few recent episodes of panic and as full an account of the first episode as it is possible to gain.

These descriptions include the circumstances in which the panic took place, the bodily reactions that were experienced, the behaviour associated with the panic, and, most importantly, the thoughts that the person had immediately before and during the episode of panic. Usually, it is possible to detect the occurrence of significant bodily sensations and associated thoughts, and to obtain an inkling of whether or not the same thoughts are repeatedly involved in the episodes.

For example, a patient whose episodes of panic appeared to occur without rhyme or reason, and in unexpected places at unexpected times, turned out to have a highly specific link between a particular bodily sensation and the experience of panic. After a close analysis that occupied four sessions and some behavioural tests, it emerged that she had experienced an inner ear infection that had seriously interfered with her balance, but this had cleared up after a course of antibiotic medication. A week later, when she was out in a shopping mall with her three young children, she had a recurrence of dizziness and fell to the ground. With assistance, she was able, gradually, to recall the thoughts that she had experienced at the time of this incident. Initially she felt that she was fainting and that there was something wrong with her brain; her anxieties turned immediately to the safety of her three children. She was frightened that if she lost consciousness, or worse, her children would be left unprotected and at risk.

In the course of the next six months she experienced eight more episodes of panic, at seemingly unconnected and inexplicable times and places, but they appeared to have a common element of feelings of dizziness or a threat of fainting, losing consciousness, or even dying. Her episodes of panic appeared to be triggered by the feelings of dizziness, sometimes even very slight feelings of which she was not fully aware; in addition, she had rapidly become sensitized to the shopping mall in which the first incident occurred, and to similar situations. She began to feel anticipatory anxiety whenever she had to re-enter the original shopping mall or others like it, which then contributed to the feelings of dizziness itself, establishing a vicious circle.

Expectations of panic

After collecting from the patient detailed descriptions of the original episode and recent panics, information is gathered about the circumstances in which attacks are most likely to occur and when they are likely to be severe. A common factor in determining the likelihood of a panic and its severity, is the presence of a trusted adult. The reasoning behind these variations in expectations of panic usually follows this pattern: 'If the pounding of my heart is an indication that I might be on the verge of a heart attack, then I am in greatest danger when alone at some distance from medical services. If, however, I am accompanied by a trusted adult, or if I am near to emergency medical services the dangers are less serious. Travelling alone to an inaccessible part of the country, especially on my own, is far too risky.'

Information is also collected about the actions or situations that might prevent an episode of panic or that would make it less severe or troubling. In addition to the presence of a trusted adult and medical services, the availability of a trusted medication may dampen down or may even prevent an episode of panic. The availability of a reliable motor vehicle helps, as does the knowledge that one's family doctor is in town and easily accessible. It is not uncommon for patients to increase their medications when their doctor is out of town.

Patients often have in-situation safety behaviour that they regularly use, and details of these are also sought. This behaviour includes, for example, tensing one's legs, holding on to solid objects like tables and railings, and sitting down if there is a fear of fainting.

Time is taken to learn about the attitudes and behaviour of other people towards the episodes of panic and especially, of course, the attitude and behaviour of close family members, employers and colleagues. It is also important to attempt to understand the patient's beliefs about the nature of the problem and what caused it.

As will be described in the section on assessment (Chapter 8), it is often useful to link the information that is collected during the clinical interview to a series of behavioural experiments. These enable the sufferer and the therapist to confirm or disconfirm whatever ideas have emerged about the underlying beliefs that are propelling the panic problem, and they frequently provide fresh information about the cognitions and other aspects of the panic episodes.

Treatment begins

Once the assessment has been completed, and some likely candidates for the source of the catastrophic thoughts have been identified, the actual treatment process begins. The therapist gives the patient a good deal of information about the nature of anxiety, episodes of panic, and the role of cognitions in causing the emotional reactions. Some patients rapidly recognize the extent to which their own experiences and thoughts fit in with this information, and find it very reassuring that their experiences are familiar, well-described, reasonably well-understood, common to many people, and responsive to treatment. The patient can change from a frightened and bewildered sufferer, tormented by a possibly sinister disorder, into a person who recognizes that they simply have a problem with controlling anxiety. Patients also welcome a form of treatment in which they take an active part with the therapist in searching for understanding and explanation, not only of their present difficulties, but of the events which led up to them. The transition from a passive sufferer, who has undergone a frightening and poorly understood series of unpredictable events, into an active searcher after the nature and causes of the problem and how to overcome them is, in almost all cases, an extremely welcome experience.

It is likely that the introductory educational part of treatment plays a major part in reassuring the patient and providing the basis on which the core of the treatment is based.

Linkages

Certain links between sensations and catastrophic thoughts are particularly common. These include: the connection between the sensation of a pounding heart and the fear of an imminent heart attack, shortness of breath and fear that one will suffocate and die, the sensation of feeling faint and the thought of passing out or dying, and unusual sensations in the head, or unusual perceptions, and the fear that one is going mad.

These links can be extremely important but they are not always obvious. Frequently patients are surprised when they learn about the strength and frequency with which they make these connections between particular sensations and specific frightening thoughts of catastrophe. Furthermore, these links between sensations and catastrophic cognitions often are associated with vivid and frightening images, as the following case studies illustrate.

 Case study

A young man complained of panics accompanied by shortness of breath and weakness in his legs. He was terrified that he would collapse and die when this happened. He had a vivid visual image, which came to him at the time, of himself lying on the ground, gasping for breath, looking hideous. Just as he began to feel the shortness of breath, the image always appeared. This unwanted and uninvited catastrophic image added to his fear and distress.

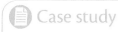
Case study

A 35-year-old female lecturer complained of a series of panics that began when her mother became seriously ill, and which then continued for over a year. The first thing that happened in her panics was feeling faint. As soon as she felt like this, she became terrified that she would die. She had a vivid image of her mother in a coffin, as she had seen her after she died, and another identical coffin, in which she could see her own 'corpse'. The image was vivid and distinct, and convinced her that she was about to drop dead. This is another example of the adverse impact of a catastrophic image.

Changing cognitions

Once the patient and therapist are reasonably sure that they have identified important links, a number of techniques are introduced that will help the person to gain more appropriate and safer interpretations of events.

These techniques include: the search for alternative explanations, considering how other people would interpret the situation, the inclusion of important facts that have been omitted or the deletion of misleading facts that are being unnecessarily included, and trying to estimate the true probability that the catastrophic event will actually take place.

'What evidence do I have for this thought?' 'Is there any alternative way of looking at the situations?' 'Is there any alternative explanation?' These questions, which are among the most commonly asked, are illustrated in the transcript below, which also highlights the value of providing information about anxiety. This transcript, from a case extract provided by Dr David Clark, is a particularly good example of the search for an alternative explanation.

Patient   'In the middle of a panic attack, I usually think I am going to faint or collapse.'

Therapist   'How much do you believe that sitting here right now, and how much would you believe it if you had the sensations you get in an attack?'

Patient   '50% now and 90% in an attack.'

Therapist   'OK, let's look at the evidence you have for this thought. Have you ever fainted in an attack?'

Patient   'No.'

Therapist   'What is it then that makes you think you might faint?'

Patient   'I feel faint and the feeling can be very strong.'

Therapist   'So, to summarize, your evidence that you are going to faint is the fact that you feel faint?'

Patient   'Yes.'

Therapist   'How can you then account for the fact that you have felt faint many hundreds of times and have not yet fainted?'

Patient   'So far, the attacks have always stopped just in time or I have managed to hold onto something to stop myself from collapsing.'

Therapist   'Right, so one explanation of the fact that you have frequently felt faint, and thought that you will faint, but have not actually fainted, is that you have always done something to save yourself just in time. However, an alternative explanation is that the feeling of faintness that you get in a panic attack will never lead you to collapsing, even if you don't control it.'

Patient   'Yes, I suppose so.'

Therapist   'In order to decide which of these possibilities is correct, we need to know what has to happen to your body for you to actually faint. Do you know?'

Patient   'No.'

Therapist   'Your blood pressure needs to drop. Do you know what happens to your blood pressure during a panic attack?'

Patient   'Well, my pulse is racing. I guess my blood pressure must be up.'

Therapist   'That's right. In anxiety, heart rate and blood pressure tend to go together. So you are actually *less* likely to faint when you are anxious than when you are not.'

Patient   'That's very interesting and helpful to know. However, if it's true, why do I feel so faint?'

Therapist   'Your feeling of faintness is a sign that your body is reacting in a normal way to the perception of danger. Most of the bodily reactions you are experiencing when anxious were probably designed to deal with the threats experienced by primitive man, such as being approached by a tiger. What would be the best thing to do in that situation?'

Patient   'Run away as fast as you can.'

Therapist   'That's right. And in order to help you run, you need the maximum amount of energy in your muscles. This is achieved by sending more of your blood to your muscles and relatively less to the brain. This means that there is a small drop in oxygen to the brain and this is why you feel faint. However, this feeling is misleading in the sense that it doesn't mean you will actually faint because your overall blood pressure is up, not down.'

Patient   'That's very clear. So next time I feel faint, I can check out whether I am going to faint by taking my pulse. If it is normal, or quicker than normal, I know I won't faint.'

Therapist   'That's right. Now, on the basis of what we've discussed so far, how much do you believe you might faint in a panic attack?'

Patient   'Less, say 10%.'

Therapist   'And if you were experiencing the sensation?'

Patient   'Maybe 25%.'

This case excerpt is from Clark (1989). Reproduced with permission.

The underlying fear of going insane is illustrated in the following case study.

 Case study

Mr S, a 35-year-old sales manager, complained of repeated episodes of panic that were distressing and also interfering with his ability to make business calls. On examination it appeared that most of the episodes of panic, and those which were near-panics, took place shortly before or at the beginning of a business call. The patient had been extremely shy as a child and had, with difficulty, gained sufficient confidence to enter business sales. It turned out that there were certain kinds of customers or settings in which he felt a surge of social anxiety and during these periods he felt extremely dizzy and felt that he was babbling incoherently. He then became extremely frightened and at times had full-blown episodes of panic. Analysis revealed that he was interpreting those periods of dizziness, and what he took to be incoherent speech, as signs that he might be having a nervous breakdown and possibly going insane. His idea of insanity, which was incorrect, had been constructed without his realizing it, on the basis of some frightening visits that he made as an adolescent to see an elderly uncle who was a long-term resident in a psychiatric hospital. The uncle suffered from chronic schizophrenia and was unresponsive for most of the time, other than making requests for cigarettes, prefaced and followed by incoherent mumbling.

When, as an adult salesman, he became socially anxious and felt that he was not speaking clearly, the patient automatically interpreted this as an early sign of impending mental illness. He then had some harrowing images of himself, disabled and deteriorated, as he had seen his uncle. With the aid of the therapist, Mr S compiled a list of the main signs of mental illness, including schizophrenia, and in another column he listed his own experiences and 'symptoms'. In the construction of this list of comparisons between the symptoms of schizophrenia and his own experiences, it became apparent that the differences were overwhelming, and gradually he lost his fear of developing schizophrenia as his uncle had done. He had no further panics, but continued to feel uneasy in awkward social situations.

It is interesting to note the effects of unwanted and uninvited images of catastrophe in this case, as in some of our other excerpts.

Behavioural experiments

The analysis and discussion of a patient's past experiences and interpretations of events is a necessary step in identifying the cognitive origin of the panics. However, the mere identification of the thoughts and attitudes may not be sufficient. Certainly, the balancing of evidence for and against a particular thought, such as the possibility of having a heart attack, may be too abstract, too removed from the actual situation to be of sufficient help. Moreover, most patients distinguish between the thoughts they have in the calm safety of the clinic, and the thoughts they have during a panic episode. In these instances, the use of so-called behavioural experiments can be extremely helpful. In addition to confirming or disconfirming the value of different sorts of evidence, they can be used to collect fresh information. And it has to be said that in many instances it is episodes of personal experience that are most effective in bringing about changes in beliefs; sometimes the patient can achieve in one successful behavioural exercise far more than hours of discussion and analysis will yield. Take the following case study example.

 ## Case study

A 25-year-old man complained of repeated episodes of panic. The episodes were severe and tended mostly to occur when he engaged in rigorous physical exercise. As a result, he had given up weight-lifting and jogging, even though he valued the exercises and regretted the decline in his physical condition that ensued when he gave up these activities. Analysis suggested that the panic episodes were generally brought on by a strong sensation of a pounding heart and oppression in the chest, which he often experienced after, or during, a strenuous session of weight-lifting (one wonders whether weight-lifting is ever not strenuous). In certain vulnerable moods he automatically interpreted the chest sensations and pounding heart as signs that he was about to have a heart attack and naturally felt extremely frightened. He reported that the episodes of panic that took place in these circumstances tended to last 15–20 minutes. In the course of a discussion about the possible interpretations of these physical sensations, the patient and therapist compiled a list of evidence supporting an interpretation that he was about to have a heart attack, versus a list of information suggesting instead that the symptoms were due to an anxious misinterpretation of the chest and heart sensations. It turned out that the patient was well aware that people who have heart conditions often experience tightness of the chest and shortness of breath as a result of vigorous exercising, but that sufferers quickly gain some relief and composure by sitting down and resting. In contrast, the same sensations that result from anxiety do not respond to the simple expedient of sitting down and resting. From his own experience, he knew that these episodes of panic, once started, tended to last from 15–20 minutes–even while resting.

In order to test these alternative interpretations, and also to give him the experience of 'surviving' a period of vigorous exercise and subsequent heart and chest sensations, a specific behavioural test was formulated. The aim was to check the effects of a period of physical rest on the patient's feelings of panic and the associated bodily sensations of chest tension and rapid heartbeat. It was agreed in advance that if the patient's unpleasant chest and heart sensations continued unchanged for up to 20 minutes after taking a rest from exercise, this result would be most consistent with the idea that the sensations were symptoms of anxiety, rather than the early signs of a heart attack. On the other hand, if they lasted for less than 20 minutes after resting, anxiety was unlikely to be the cause.

The behavioural test was duly carried out on two separate occasions. The first attempt to induce panicky feelings during vigorous physical exercise that included weight-lifting proved to be unsuccessful. The patient had become aware that he was sweating and that his heart had increased its rate, but there were no alarming physical sensations and it was therefore impossible to test the effects of the pre-arranged rest period. On the second attempt, however, about 20 minutes into the vigorous exercising he began to be alarmed by feelings of pressure in his chest and by a racing heart. As on a number of previous episodes, he began to feel panicky and to think that he might be in the early stages of a heart attack. Fortunately, he was nevertheless able to carry out the test as planned. He sat down in a comfortable chair for 30 minutes, and found that the uncomfortable sensations and panicky feelings persisted unchanged for 18 minutes before entering a slow decline. Even though he was resting, the cardiac sensations persisted.

When the results of the two tests were discussed, the patient concluded that they were more consistent with the interpretation that he was experiencing anxiety rather than an imminent heart attack. The behavioural tests also gave rise to a memory that he felt was relevant. Apparently he had heard about a year ago that an elderly uncle of one of his acquaintances had had a serious heart attack while exercising at a local gymnasium. Furthermore, he was able to remember that, during a number of panic episodes associated with exercising, he had definitely had thoughts and images of the old man suddenly being struck down by a heart attack.

Patients whose panicky thoughts incorporate a fear of imminent medical catastrophe, such as a heart attack, readily agree that their panicky feelings decrease when they are distracted. The question is: Can anyone distract oneself from a heart attack, or other catastrophes, such as brain tumours or loss of consciousness? The effects of distraction can provide the basis for valuable experiments on the patients' fears and reactions.

Dealing with images

It is not uncommon for patients with panic disorder to experience repetitive, intrusive, stereotyped images, which add to their distress. In some, these images are a key factor that contributes to, and worsens, the panic. The images can contribute to the person's fear of a catastrophic event, and even trigger a panic. One patient reported a vivid image of lying on the roadside after an accident, in a state of collapse, with blood coming from her mouth. Another had a recurrent image of being trapped in an abandoned tunnel.

It has been found that many of these images have their origin in some distressing event during childhood. Not infrequently the frightening images arise out of catastrophic events that occurred to other people, especially to family members or friends. Examples of this type, referred to earlier, include the person who was tormented by a recurring image of her father's death, and another who was distressed and alarmed by the image of a relation who had been disfigured by a stroke. Some intrusive images arise indirectly, out of catastrophic events that the person has read about or heard about, for example airline accidents.

The images are intrusive, unwanted, vivid, fully formed, do not change over time, are distressing, and strongly resisted. As a result, the affected person struggles to block or wipe out the images, but this can be extremely difficult, and the person may need professional help.

In many cases the images can be dealt with by using the usual cognitive methods and behavioural experiments, described in the previous sections. However, in some cases the addition of specific imagery techniques is necessary and effective. One technique is to 'finish out' the image; i.e. to imagine what would happen next, beyond the frozen image reflecting catastrophe. One aim of this tactic is to promote a sense of control over the alarming image. A related technique involves helping the patient to restructure, or transform, the image.

For example, a patient with a frightening image of herself lying on the floor in a crowded supermarket may be helped to transform it so that she now imagines herself getting up safely with the help of a bystander, thanking this person with a smile, and walking away. The patient needs to rehearse the new imagery sequence with the help of the therapist. This kind of specific imagery work can play a useful part in the therapy.

Overcoming avoidance behaviour

As described earlier, the main weapon against excessive avoidance behaviour is the introduction of planned and methodical exposure exercises. To some extent, these exposure exercises also function as behavioural tests in that some of the person's maladaptive cognitions are challenged and disconfirmed during the conduct of the exercises. For example, the idea that one might become dizzy and then faint on a bus can be put to repeated behavioural tests by planned journeys on selected bus routes, usually starting with the easiest journey and the least crowded buses, and then progressively moving towards more difficult bus rides. The patient learns that, even if they do experience sensations of faintness, these never progress to the point of losing consciousness. Plainly, if one persistently avoids going on the bus, the belief that the sensations of faintness are a sure sign of an impending loss of consciousness will never be tested, and hence can not be disconfirmed.

Changes during treatment: an example

A large majority of people benefit from psychological therapy. Those who do not may be suffering from a related problem that impedes progress, such as depression, or the failure to improve may be due to other reasons. The personal account given below, from a senior professional person whose panics reduced her to a nearly housebound life, conveys the changes during treatment.

 ## Patient's perspective

It's been about 13 months since you 'let me loose', so I thought I'd let you know how I was doing. I will always remember my first day in your consulting room when I just sat and cried because my world was so small because of my panic disorder. I had gone from being a person who had never thought about whether I could or could not do anything, regardless of the complexity of the task (I just did it), to one who at times couldn't even leave my house. On that day, when I said I would not allow this to control my life, I remember you told me that panic disorder was an entirely treatable condition and that I was going to be alright. For the first time, despite my own personal doubts, you gave me hope that there was light at the end of the tunnel. Although I couldn't see that light … just the overwhelming darkness of the tunnel …

My road to recovery was long and hard, but you know what, I made it! Every time, I took a slide backwards, I managed to climb back up the ladder of recovery and reached a level at least two rungs higher than where I had been before.

I have learned to pace myself, delegate, perhaps guide people how to solve their problems, but not to do it for them. I have learned that it's OK not to be perfect. As you know, I held myself to a different yardstick than I did for the others around me. Every once in a while, I find myself falling into my old habits but I have also learned to say 'No'. All in all, I have learned while it's OK to take care of other people, first of all you have to take care of yourself.

Every once in a while when I am crossing a bridge, standing in a line up or in a crowded room, I will become somewhat awe-struck. I remember when all of those simple things were so hard, and at times impossible, for me to do. I remember feeling like I was one of Pavlov's dogs and unable to get out of the cage created by my disorder. I remember how I used to cry often when I saw a 7–11 store because I thought that if I was able to reach a level where I could work again, that working in 7–11 was going to be the highest I would be able to achieve. I remember at times being in the depths of despair because of the seemingly insurmountable limitations imposed by my disorder.

Work is going great. As you know, in order to return to work, I had to initially agree to assume all of the responsibilities that I had prior to my leave of absence, inclusive of flying around the country at ungodly hours of the day and night. My initial intent was to stay for 6 months in order to cross the hurdles I knew I had to cross and then get the heck out of there. I was so scared going back. My department had deteriorated into a horrible mess in my absence. The staff was on the edge of breakdown because of overwork.

Within six months, I persuaded the administration to let me hire more staff. I developed a work rotation that would allow my staff to take time off in lieu of the massive amounts of overtime that they work. Initially my staff, who are all type A personalities like myself, were resistant to taking the time off, but I forced them to do it. I gave them a vivid picture of what it was like to have no groceries at home but to be too terrified to make the simple steps of getting into the car and going to the grocery store. They are learning to pace themselves. The administration and myself have seen the remarkable transition in my department from being very dysfunctional to relatively happy, productive, and rested.

I have been able to cross almost every hurdle that I had to face. It wasn't easy but I did it. The one thing that has taken the longest is speaking in front of others. I had been an accomplished public speaker prior to all this happening. I joined Toastmasters and have been working hard on getting that back. When I gave my first speech (in which you are supposed to let the group get to know you), I spoke about my trials and tribulations with panic disorder and my struggle back … I got a standing ovation.

I used to look at panic disorder as a personal failure. I thought that because of it, I had lost over two years of my life. Gradually, I have come to think of it as a gift from God… it was a wake-up call to change my ways or else. Because of my panic disorder, I am a better person in all regards.

So, I just thought I'd let you know about a success story. And remember … don't work too hard … life is just too short.

Relapse prevention

The development of depression, or ill-health, or a period of exceptional stress, can cause a return of the fear. If the patient was treated with medications, a resumption of the drugs may suffice to diminish the panics. If not, attempts will be made to find a suitable alternative medication.

Patients who receive psychological treatment are given advice about the possibility of a return of the fear, and how to manage it. In order to prevent a relapse from occurring, the closing sessions of treatment become increasingly educational. These sessions are widely spaced, and patients are encouraged to take on more and more of the planning and conduct of the treatment so that they can become independent, and gain increasing self-confidence about their ability to deal with, and control, the problem unassisted. Patients are also given advice about circumstances in which recurrences might occur, such as fresh stresses or conflicts, losses or bereavements, depression, episodes of ill-health, the emergence of new catastrophic cognitions, and so forth. Some time is spent in going over how the patient can recognize the signs of a possible return of panic, and what they should do to prevent it from recurring. For example: 'If you notice that you are becoming increasingly sensitive to your heart beat and starting to have frightening ideas or images, restart your daily recordings and try to find what, if anything, is triggering the thoughts and images. Once you have that information, set down the evidence for and against at least two alternative interpretations, and then proceed to test them. If you find yourself starting to avoid situations for reasons of fear, that is the surest sign that you need to enter those situations repeatedly, and remain there for increasing periods of time.'

Patients are encouraged to continue using the methods acquired during treatment as a means of protecting and promoting their feelings of control and self-confidence. For example, they are encouraged to practice their anti-avoidance behaviour by deliberately going into those places and situations that formerly scared them. They are encouraged to recognize and dismiss any panic cognitions that pop-up, and dismiss any unadaptive interpretations of their bodily sensations and panic images.

Patients whose original problems included sustained and extensive avoidance should be advised of the need to continue practising their behavioural exercises, even after treatment has been completed. The original fear and avoidance can creep back gradually and the best way to prevent a troublesome return of these fears is to 'keep psychologically fit', in a manner that resembles physical fitness. If runners, sportspeople, athletes neglect exercising, they lose their feelings of fitness and strength. Similarly, people who have overcome their fearful avoidance should keep fit by taking reasonable practice—keep going out, using public transport, shopping, driving, going to crowded places, and so forth.

Patients are told that if the problem becomes unmanageable, they are welcome to seek further assistance, and reminded that booster or retreatment sessions are generally successful and require comparatively few visits. For many patients, the mere knowledge that the channels remain open is sufficient to provide that degree of security that enables them to manage largely unassisted.

How effective is psychological treatment?

Reviewing the results of several scientific investigations of the effects of cognitive therapy, one of the pioneers of this type of treatment, Dr David Clark of the London University, concluded that an average of 84% of patients with panic disorder are free of panics after therapy (12–15 sessions, but for some with as few as 6 sessions). When they were assessed for follow-up, ranging from 3 to 12 months, the percentage of panic-free patients stood at 78. The results were reassuringly lasting, consistent across clinics, and indeed across countries; the studies were carried out in the UK, USA, Holland, Sweden, and Germany. The NICE evaluations of psychological treatment are favourable, and cognitive behaviour therapy is strongly recommended because the effects are substantial and endure longer than the results of other treatments.

An important advantage of psychological treatment is that there are no side-effects to contend with, and no dietary or other restrictions.

Group treatment is feasible and reasonably effective.

Combined psychological and pharmacological treatment

A number of attempts have been made to combine psychological treatment and medication in the hope of producing stronger effects. This is a plausible expectation but a combination of the two methods rarely produces results that are superior to each type of therapy used separately. There is some concern about whether or not the tendency to relapse when medication is stopped might also have an adverse effect on the psychological treatment. The available evidence suggests that this can be avoided if the drug is withdrawn slowly and carefully.

The results of an unusually large study, carried out by Dr David Barlow of Boston University and three colleagues from Pittsburgh, New York and New Haven, confirmed that medication and psychological therapy are effective, but there were few signs that a combination of these two types of therapy produces a superior outcome. A total of 312 patients were given medication (imipramine) or cognitive-behaviour therapy, or a combination of both types of treatment. At the end of the therapy period it was found that imipramine and cognitive-behaviour therapy both produced significant, and approximately equal, improvements. These improvements were superior to those seen after treatment with the inert medication (placebo) that was included for purposes of comparison. There was a higher relapse rate for patients who were medicated (25%) than for those who had cognitive-behaviour therapy (4%). The psychological treatment was well tolerated and its effects were durable, but it required more time and effort.

In practice, large numbers of patients receive a combination of psychological and pharmacological treatments. There appears to be little reason for concern about the combination, assuming it is sensibly done. Equally, there is so far no compelling evidence that the combination leads to major advantages. In those cases where drug treatment has been used initially with beneficial effect, following on with some psychological treatment is likely to reduce the chances of relapse.

Treatment of panic disorder that is associated with other psychological problems

In many cases of panic disorder, the person is also affected by one or more other psychological problems, notably social anxiety, depression, generalized anxiety disorder, obsessive–compulsive disorder. This type of association is called 'co-morbidity', and not infrequently it complicates the treatment of panic disorders. The following examples illustrate how interactions between the panic and the associated problems can cause complications.

There is a close relation between panic and depression. As many as 50% of patients with panic disorder have concurrent depression or antecedant depression. If a patient receiving therapy for panic is simultaneously suffering from clinical depression, the analysis of the relevant cognitions tends to be blurred by the interaction between the panic cognitions and those that are part of the depression. Progress in dealing with the disturbing cognitions can be slowed down, and, in addition, the patient may find that his persistently negative mood and low energy preclude carrying out the behavioural exercises that are necessary. These obstacles can be reduced by the addition of anti-depressant medication.

When the panics are associated with obsessive–compulsive disorder, particularly if the patient is burdened by intense fears of contamination, treatment is complicated. In most cases, the therapist first tackles the fear of contamination by psychological therapy, and when the fear diminishes sufficiently, shifts the focus to treating the panics. This sequence is used when the fear of contamination drives extensive avoidance, and when unpredicted or unavoidable contacts with a contaminant provoke episodes of panic. Attempting to treat the panics without first reducing the fears of contamination can be difficult.

If the panic disorder is associated with intense social anxiety, a comparable sequence may be utilized in which the patient begins with cognitive behaviour therapy for the cognitions and unadaptive social behaviour, and the emphasis later changes to dealing directly with the panics. This sequence is selected if the person is experiencing panics in stressful social situations.

Diagnostically it is sometimes difficult to distinguish between panic disorder and generalized anxiety disorder (GAD). Panic disorder is characterized by recurrent episodes of unexpected panic and associated situational panics. The main features of GAD are chronic anxiety and exaggerated worries about realistic, even minor, matters. Affected patients are restless, troubled, over-aroused, and over-vigilant. They are regarded as 'worriers'. If the patient is burdened by panic and by chronic worries cognitive behaviour therapy is effective but can be complicated and lengthy.

Group treatment

Group treatment is an economic alternative to individual psychological treatment, and the results of the two forms are equivalent. Group treatment (5–8 patients, weekly sessions for 8–10 weeks) has some advantages, such as group exposure exercises, but it is not suitable for complex or severe cases.

Computer-assisted treatment

Some progress has been made in producing computer programs that enable people to understand and better deal with their panics and agoraphobic avoidance, but the results are not consistent. Some people make substantial progress but others find the programs unhelpful. It is probable that improved programs will enable many people to overcome the worst of their problems, especially if they fall into the mild to moderate category. In severe cases computer-assisted programs are unlikely to be effective.

Treatments that are not recommended

The authoritative NICE evaluations of treatments for panic disorder/agoraphobia span a wide range, and some methods are explicitly discounted. Among others, the following methods are not recommended: hypnosis, psychoanalysis, psychodynamic therapy, muscle relaxation, eye-movement desensitization and reprocessing (EMDR), neurolinguistic programming.

Severe cases

The results of large-scale treatment trials have not shown that the initial severity of person's panic disorder, with or without agoraphobia, has much influence on the successful outcome of therapy. However, in clinical practice it is difficult to treat some of the severe cases, not least because their very disorder prevents them from attending therapy on a regular basis, and/or carrying out the recommended 'homework exposure-exercises'. A small number are virtually housebound. It is possible that because of their extreme difficulties, severely affected patients are not fully represented in conventional treatment trials, and hence it has not been shown that initial severity has an influence on outcome. In severe cases medication is often used to relieve distress and facilitate psychological treatment.

Self-help organizations have been established during the past few years and the best of them are invaluable for sufferers and their friends and relatives. They are a source of extensive and helpful information–about the disorder, drugs, recent developments, self-help groups, and local therapists and services. The group members can be a valuable source of emotional support, understanding and encouragement.

Details of some of these organizations are given in Appendix 4.

Self-help groups can be a source of unmatched empathy, comfort, and special understanding. They can also serve as a medium for treatment, especially for isolated people, and are an unrivalled source of information about treatment facilities, medications, therapists, and so on.

Some of the self-help organizations, including many listed in Appendix 4, provide advice about forming and running self-help groups.

7

Further aspects of treatment

→ Key Points

- After the initial episode of panic, a full medical examination is desirable in order to assess the person's health status.

- In the absence of any significant and relevant health problems, little action is likely to follow.

- After a second and subsequent panics, referral to a clinical psychologist or psychiatrist is considered.

- A diagnosis of panic disorder will be made if repeated episodes of panic, persisting anxiety and developing avoidance behaviour, are evident.

- Depending on the individual case a recommendation for medication and/or psychological therapy will be made.

Primary care of panic disorders

During the first experience of panic, especially if it occurs unexpectedly, it is common for people to seek medical help. In many cases the person goes to, or is transported to, an emergency medical facility, particularly if they feel in danger of having a heart attack. The young woman described on p.2, who experienced chest pains and breathing difficulties, felt that she was having a heart attack, and her husband rushed her to the nearest hospital emergency clinic. After a full examination, the doctors reassured her that her heart was entirely normal, and she went home feeling shaken but relieved. When, a few days later, she had her second panic, she realized that a serious and puzzling health problem had emerged and consulted her family doctor.

In the early stages of the disorder, sufferers from unrecognized panic disorder will do the same as anyone facing a serious imminent threat to their health—urgently seek medical care. After the first one or two episodes of panic, it becomes clear that the problem cannot be dealt with by visits to the emergency clinic of a hospital. It is common at this stage to visit one's family doctor, who may deal with the problem. However, if the problem is not resolved at this facility, a referral to a specialist service, such as a clinical psychologist or a psychiatrist, may follow.

Patients who consult their family doctor after episodes of intense fear accompanied by disturbing bodily sensations and a sense of impending catastrophe may be suffering from one of a variety of problems other than panic disorder. After the doctor successfully rules out the other possibilities, attention is paid to specific episodes and the presence or absence of additional stresses in the two months prior to the first episode.

A diagnosis of panic disorder is made if the patient has had repeated episodes of panic within the past month or two, at least some of which were 'spontaneous' and were followed by prolonged feelings of anxiety and apprehension. The emergence of avoidance behaviour is a confirming feature.

The family doctor will assess the presence/absence of previous periods of anxiety, and collect information about recent stressful events or anticipated events, and their possible relation to the panics. Because of the common association of panic with depression, the assessment will include a search for signs of depression (feelings of helplessness, despair, crying, insomnia, loss of energy/interest). Patients with panic disorder report intense fear when they feel short of breath, and/or feel faint, and/or feel shaky, and/or their heart beats rapidly.

If a diagnosis is made of panic disorder, the family doctor can provide information and reassuring explanations, supplemented, if possible, by reading materials. The patient will also be encouraged to attempt to maintain their normal daily activities and to 'avoid avoidance'. Depending on the severity and frequency of the panics and anxiety, medication may or may not be prescribed. If the panics and/or anxiety and avoidance persist and are distressing or disabling, specialist treatment may be required.

With the rolling introduction of massively increased numbers of psychological therapists, and the provision of a self-referral system that enables people to make direct arrangements with their local psychological service, it should be possible to obtain timely assistance. Many people who start experiencing sudden, inexplicable panics will continue to consult their family doctor as the first resource.

Hyperventilation (over-breathing)

Disturbed breathing is a typical response to a threatening event (such as an unexplained noise late at night) and, as already noted, feeling short of breath is a common experience during panic episodes. In fact, shortness of breath is one of the four most commonly reported panic sensations; the other three are: rapid heart beat, sweating, and dizziness. People who frequently experience fearful feelings of shortness of breath tend to take precautionary measures; they prefer open windows, even in cold weather, avoid stale air, stuffy rooms, and so forth.

A patient who feared a sudden heart attack experienced numerous panics during which his breathing became shallow and rapid, and made him gasp for air. He became particularly sensitive to fresh air. On numerous occasions he fully opened all of the windows of his car when driving in severe winter weather. A school-teacher who had a similar problem with over-breathing insisted on keeping open the windows of his classrooms, even during winter. This habit was not popular with his pupils.

Hyperventilation can be a contributing cause of a panic episode, or merely one feature of the episode, albeit an intense and distressing one. Rapid, shallow breathing can produce a number of disturbing bodily reactions, such as light-headedness, rapid heart beat, tingling in the fingers and toes, pressure in the chest, and a flushed face. These sensations are unpleasant in themselves, but they can also lead to a full-blown panic.

If the person makes a catastrophic misinterpretation of these unwanted sensations, a panic can occur. Such common misinterpretations include: 'I feel light-headed and dizzy, and am about to lose consciousness or lose control', 'My heart is pounding, and that means I am in danger of straining my heart and dying', and 'The pressure in my chest is a symptom of an oncoming heart attack'.

Hyperventilation tests

In the assessment phase, patients may be asked to undertake a brief test in order to determine whether or not hyperventilation is playing a part in the episodes of panic. The reason for, and the nature of, the test is explained in order to obtain the patient's informed consent and co-operation. A typical test takes place as follows:

Typical test for hyperventilation

'I would like you to carry out a short, simple test of your breathing. When I ask you to begin, please start breathing shallowly and rapidly, and continue to do so until I ask you to stop at the end of two minutes. If you wish to do so, you can of course, stop at any time, but do try to continue for the full two minutes if you can.'

'Before we begin, please tell me if you are at all anxious at present. Use a 0–100 scale, a sort of thermometer of anxiety, in which 0 is completely calm and 100 is terror. You can use any part of the scale, so 20/100 would indicate very slight anxiety, 50/100 moderate anxiety, 80/100 intense fear, and so on. What is your score at present, out of 100?'

'Are you aware of any bodily sensations at present?'

After ensuring that the patient understands the instructions, the therapist begins the test.

'Now begin over-breathing and try to continue until I tell you that the two minutes are up. Please go ahead.'

Sometimes it is necessary for the therapist to demonstrate the over-breathing exercise in order to make sure the patient understands what is needed.

At the end of the test period the patient re-rates his/her anxiety, 0–100, and is also asked to describe any new or persisting bodily sensations. Commonly the test result is positive and the patient recognizes that some of the feelings resemble those that they have experienced during episodes of panic. One patient observed, 'It was very similar to how I feel during a panic, but somehow less real, less frightening'.

The results of the hyperventilation test can be revealing, as in the following case study.

 Case study

A 42-year-old woman had repeatedly experienced intense episodes of panic. During the hyperventilation test she initially became very dizzy and light-headed, and those reactions then developed into a major panic. It turned out that the dizziness, light-headedness, and pressure she felt in her head during the over-breathing triggered a thought that she had something wrong in her brain. Further analysis revealed that the underlying, terrifying thought was that she had a cancerous tumour in the brain. Eight years earlier, she had undergone surgery for the successful removal of a cancerous tumour of the breast, but was plagued by fears of a recurrence of the cancer in other parts of her body. (Her mother and a maternal aunt had both died of secondary cancers.) One of the major causes of her panics was a catastrophic misinterpretation of the sensations produced by spontaneous over-breathing, and she subsequently derived relief from a recognition of this connection, and a course of breathing retraining.

People who habitually hyperventilate can learn to regulate and control their breathing. With practice, they acquire the ability to impose a slow, steady rhythm on their breathing at will, reducing the tendency to over-breathe. For some, the use of a small paper bag proves helpful. The effects of over-breathing, including the unpleasant associated sensations, are sometimes reversible within minutes of breathing into a paper bag that fits over the nose and mouth.

It is not known for certain why some people habitually over-breathe, but at least two contributing factors have been identified. Firstly, people who have had some respiratory illness or difficulties (such as asthma) may be at some risk of over-breathing. Secondly, people who have an intense fear of suffocation are also inclined to over-breathe, perhaps in compensation for their worries about not getting sufficient air into their lungs.

In many cases there is a connection between panic disorder and the fear of suffocation, which can provide the basis for episodes of panic: any threat to one's air supply, whether a true threat or a catastrophic misinterpretation of events, can provoke a panic. Hence, people who strongly fear suffocation are at an increased risk for panic when they find themselves in a small, enclosed space. It is just the setting in which a panic can occur. Indeed, in laboratory research one of the most reliable ways of provoking mild panics is by asking people to remain for a few minutes in a small enclosure such as a kiosk or chamber.

Hyperventilation tests: a caution

It is important to stress that hyperventilation tests should not be attempted in certain medical conditions. These include: epilepsy, hypertension, hypotension, asthma and other respiratory diseases, and cardiovascular illness. They should not be performed during pregnancy.

Breathing retraining

Breathing retraining, which is often incorporated into a general course of relaxation training, is useful in the treatment of panic disorder particularly if the patient is prone to hyperventilate. The aim of the training is to teach the person to adopt a slow, paced rate of breathing at will, and to use the method whenever they begin to over-breathe.

Patients are taught to breathe smoothly and slowly, reducing the rate from 16 to 20 breaths per minute to roughly 8 breaths per minute. After observing the rate and pattern of the patient's breathing, the therapist begins to pace it.

'Now that you are in a comfortable, relaxed position, please concentrate on your breathing. Take a deep breath in through your nose … fill your lungs… good, now hold that for one second … and now release all the air. Expel it all, and release any tension in your body as you expel the air.'

'Now, once again fill your lungs … take a slow deep breath … hold it … now release, let it all go.'

'Breathe in … hold it … release it.'

After a few minutes of slow, paced breathing the therapist encourages the patient to repeat the instructions to themselves: 'Now I would like you to repeat to yourself the breathing instructions. Keep to a regular, rhythmic pattern. Breathe in … hold it … breathe out … breathe in … breathe out.'

'From now on, try to control your own breathing in this way, whenever the need arises.'

Patients learn the method easily and quickly, and commonly find that it relieves tension and adds to a general feeling of relaxation. They are encouraged to use slow, paced breathing in their everyday activities, especially if they start over-breathing and/or feeling the bodily sensations that are part of their pattern of panics. They are also encouraged to think of paced, slow breathing as a means of controlling their otherwise unruly, troubling reactions.

Other methods of breathing training have also been recommended by therapists. One such method is increasing the movement of the diaphragm, especially during inhalation.

It should be noted that within the recent past some scientists have advised a reconsideration of the value of breathing retraining. Their concern is that the use of such exercises may inadvertently reinforce the (false) idea that patients are in danger and need to take steps to ensure their own safety. Until the matter is resolved breathing retraining will continue to feature in most treatment programmes.

Treating children and adolescents

In the psychological treatment of panic disorder in child and adolescent patients, the principles used in treating adults are applicable, although with young children the cognitive part of the therapy may not be possible or feasible in its full extent. What is particularly important in the management of these patients is enlisting the support, co-operation and involvement of the family in the treatment. Liaison with the child's school might be necessary.

8

Assessment and evaluation

Key Points

- A full assessment of the problem is necessary for diagnosis, planning of treatment, and evaluation of treatment.

- The assessment includes comprehensive interviews, psychological tests and behavioral observations.

- Some of the common tests are described, and reproduced in part.

- During the course of treatment the patient is encouraged to maintain a simple daily record of panic episodes and related events; the non-occurrence of expected panics is as important as the panic episodes.

- Physiological testing is occasionally used in assessing panic disorder but does not form part of the standard assessment.

- There are no laboratory tests for panic disorder.

Aims of assessment

Assessment is carried out to determine the nature of the problem, and to make a diagnosis. Later, in the course of treatment, assessments are undertaken to evaluate progress. The criteria used in the diagnosis of panic disorder were described in Chapter 1, and seldom present a major problem. The criteria are set out clearly and the necessary information can be collected without difficulty: the occurrence of repeated episodes of intense fear of sudden onset, some of which are unexpected and which peak within minutes, accompanied by a number of bodily sensations. The episodes of panic are followed by a period of worry, and often lead to the development of avoidance behaviour. The diagnostic problems that do arise generally concern the coexistence of other disorders, and the relationship between these and the panic disorder itself. For example, it is sometimes difficult to disentangle the interactions between panic and depression. Once the diagnosis is established, more detailed assessments are undertaken in order to collect information for devising a treatment programme.

Methods of assessment

Interview

The main method of assessment is the clinical interview, which may take up to two hours to complete and is sometimes spread over more than one session. The patient is asked for full details of the problem, and especially how and when the first panic occurred. It also covers the way in which it affects their work, social life, and relationships. Questions will be asked about how and when it all started and what the course of the disorder has been, including fluctuations in severity, relation to stressful events, and so on. Most clinicians follow one of the standardized procedures for carrying out such interviews.

It is particularly important for purposes of the original diagnosis, and for the later evaluation, to have a full and clear description of the original and the most recent episodes of panic. The patient is asked to describe these panics in considerable detail. Some of the key details are reflected in the following questions: Where did it happen? Were you aware of any bodily sensations? What were they? How intense was the fear? What did you think was happening to you? What action did you take, if any? Did it come on you suddenly? How long did it last? Do you have any ideas about what caused it?

An attempt is then made to find out whether the early and recent episodes are similar, or whether they have changed, and it is also important to gain some idea as to whether the episodes being described are typical or unusual. Next, attention is turned to the immediate consequences of the episode of panic: What further action did you take? How did you feel at the end of the episode? What happened on the following and subsequent days? What did you think was happening to you?

Information is then collected about the longer term consequences of the episodes of panic with particular attention to what avoidance behaviour, if any, has been generated by the episodes of panic. During the interview the patient is asked about factors or activities that may prevent or dampen an episode of panic, and what factors appear to precipitate or intensify the episodes of panic.

It is particularly important to get a clear idea of the person's understanding of the nature and cause of the episodes of panic. The therapist will ask several questions in an attempt to elucidate this.

Information will also be collected about the personal and family history of the patient. Particular attention must be paid to collecting information about the person's health, and whether any past illnesses feature in the thoughts that are associated with the panics (such as a history of respiratory illnesses, a fear of suffocation during panic). The health history of members of the family and, where relevant, of close friends should be noted. In many instances the person's interpretation of what is happening during the episode of panic is coloured by their knowledge of the illnesses of relatives or friends.

Given the close and common association between panic disorder and depression, the therapist will ask several questions to find out if the person is currently suffering from a significant depression, or has done so in the past, focusing on the two main elements of clinical depression: one pertaining to feelings of subjective sadness, helplessness, and worthlessness; and a second feature concerning changes in bodily functions, such as insomnia, loss of appetite, loss of sexual drive, and loss of energy.

It is common to record the assessment interviews, if the patient agrees. Transcripts of the interviews are a valuable record and enable the therapist to monitor how changes take place over time. For example, it is useful to examine how the patient's understanding of the nature and causes of panic attacks has changed after, say, eight sessions of therapy.

Interviewing others

In many cases it is useful to interview a family member or friend as part of the assessment. Some aspects of the patient's problems can be more clearly described by a family member than by the patient; for example, the problems and stresses caused by the patient's demands and avoidance behaviour may be minimized in the patient's own account. The full extent of the patient's avoidance behaviour may not become apparent until the information is completed by another person. Most therapists will want to interview a key informant as an essential part of the assessment. In the case of children and adolescents, interviewing parents/guardians is, of course, an indispensable part of the assessment.

Behavioural tests and direct observation

Sometimes a therapist may carry out one or more behavioural tests with a patient, most commonly to get some idea of the person's range of mobility, and the probability of an episode being provoked in particular settings. The patient's reactions during these test excursions will often provide important information; e.g. How long can the patient stay in a crowded supermarket without feeling the urge to escape? What physical sensations are reported while they are there? And, what thoughts are reported as going through their mind? These 'real-life' assessments are relatively easy to set up, and many clinicians include them in their assessment routine.

Subjective ratings

The therapist is likely to ask the patient to give subjective ratings of fear. Examples were given in Chapter 6 of hierarchies of feared situations used in behavioural therapy. These hierarchies, or lists of events in order of difficulty, are usually constructed on the basis of the patient's ratings of anxiety. The most commonly used rating scale is 0–100, where 0 means no fear at all, and 100 means absolute terror. It is described to the patient as a sort of 'fear thermometer'. Patients find this type of scale easy to use. In the assessment of panic disorder, the clinician may ask the patient to give such ratings for: fear, urge to flee, probability of a severe panic, strength of various beliefs (such as the strength of the belief that the panic is a sign of serious heart disease). These ratings are also illustrated in the excerpt from Dr David Clark's interview with a patient given on pp.51–53.

Physiological tests

The direct observation of a person during a test walk or other excursion can be supplemented by the collection of physiological information, most often a recording of the person's heart rate. During most episodes of panic the patient's heart rate increases by anything from 3 to 25 beats per minute. When this happens, it is useful to know whether the increase in heart rate precedes or follows the person's feelings of fear and the accompanying thoughts. Physiological tests can be useful in assessing therapeutic progress. Physiological recording is not routinely carried out in most clinics, but some clinicians do include this in their assessment procedure.

Record keeping

It is common for the therapist to ask the patient to keep a daily record of the occurrence of anxiety and/or panic for a week or two prior to starting the active therapy, in order to establish a baseline against which to measure later progress. The most common record is a simple weekly diary in which the person records on each day the degree of anxiety that they experienced, and the occurrence or non-occurrence of episodes of panic. The panic episodes are described briefly in a separate record with a note of the intensity and duration of the episode and accompanying sensations and thoughts. An example of a diary is given in Figure 8.1, and a record of panic episodes is shown in Figure 8.2. As can be seen, the record focuses on specific problems.

Week commencing:

Day	Highest anxiety (0–100)	Number of panics (if any)
Monday		
Tuesday		
Wednesday		
Thursday		
Friday		
Saturday		
Sunday		

Figure 8.1 A blank example of a weekly diary.

Date:
Time:
Place:
Alone or accompanied:
If accompanied, by whom:
Activity at the time:
Duration:
Expected or unexpected:
Maximum anxiety felt (0–100):
Physical sensations:
Thoughts:
Outcome – what happened in the end?

Figure 8.2 A blank example of a record of panic episodes.

A simply structured weekly diary is easier to use and more meaningful to analyse than unstructured, haphazard accounts. The same applies to the record of panics. These records provide a measure of progress, as well as keeping the patient and the therapist informed of any changes in the nature or circumstances of the episodes of panic. The information gathered in the diary and the panic record often helps to clarify the causes, events, or activities that have been contributing to the panics.

Examples of a completed diary and a completed record of panics are given in Figures 8.3 and 8.4, respectively.

Week commencing: 3 October

Day	Highest anxiety (0–100)	Number of panics (if any)
Monday	70	1
Tuesday	40	0
Wednesday	45	0
Thursday	70	0
Friday	35	0
Saturday	85	1
Sunday	25	0

Figure 8.3 A completed example of a weekly diary.

Date:	8th October
Time:	About 11.30 a.m.
Place:	Post office
Alone or accompanied:	Alone
If accompanied, by whom:	——
Activity at the time:	Waiting in queue
Duration:	About 2–3 minutes
Expected or unexpected:	Unexpected
Maximum anxiety felt (0–100):	70
Physical sensations:	Shortness of breath, dizziness, sweating, feeling weak, feeling about to fall
Thoughts:	I am going to collapse here. I will make a fool of myself. What if I die here.
Outcome – what happened in the end?	Held on to the railing and steadied myself. Then managed to walk out of the building. Got some fresh air. It was okay then. But I did not go back into the post office.

Figure 8.4 A completed example of a record of panic episodes.

Questionnaires and inventories

Standard questionnaires are also used for assessment. Indeed, many therapists use them as a routine part of the assessment procedure. They have the advantage of covering a range of difficulties and facilitating the collection of a good deal of information rapidly. They also yield a numerical summary score that can be used in a screening procedure and to get a broad view of progress. The responses to the questionnaires supplement the information collected during the interview.

The most commonly used instrument with panic disorder patients is the Mobility Inventory, which was briefly mentioned in Chapter 4, and is reproduced in Appendix 1. It consists of 26 items and yields an overall score, plus details about the activities which cause particular problems for the patient in question. A rating on a 5-point scale, from 1 (never avoid) to 5 (always avoid), is given by the patient for a variety of places or situations. There are separate ratings for avoidance when alone and avoidance when accompanied by a trusted companion. A second questionnaire is the Cognitions Questionnaire, the purpose of which is to obtain some introductory information about the types of frightening thoughts the person might be experiencing. Many of the items of this questionnaire were cited in Chapter 2 (see Table 2.1). The patient rates each of 14 items to indicate the frequency with which each thought occurred when they were anxious. The ratings are from 1 (thought never occurs) to 5 (thought always occurs). The full questionnaire is given in Appendix 2.

As treatment progresses, the instruments can be re-administered to track whether the original avoidance behaviour and fearful thoughts persist or are changing.

These two questionnaires are often supplemented by a questionnaire that screens for the presence or absence of depression, most commonly the Beck Depression Inventory. This consists of 21 items and yields an overall score that ranges from 0 to 63. The items cover areas such as sadness, sex drive, appetite, energy, sleep, feelings of guilt, feeling ugly, crying, suicidal thoughts, and so on. For each item, a group of four statements is given, and the patient chooses one or more of these as reflecting how they have been in the week up to the day of completing the questionnaire. The statements carry a score of 0, 1, 2, or 3. The score of the chosen statement (or the highest one, if more than one is chosen) is counted towards the overall score. Scores above 10 are taken as indicating the presence of mild depression, scores above 16 indicating moderate depression, and scores above 25 indicating severe depression. These cut-off points are not absolute and are used as a rough guide. Like the other scales, the Beck Depression Inventory is re-administered at various times in the course of treatment to track the persistence or changes in the patient's depression.

It must be noted that, while these are the most commonly used in the assessment of panic disorder patients, there are other questionnaires and inventories that are popular with some therapists. The Anxiety Sensitivity Index is an instrument now used by many. This consists of 16 items and it measures sensitivity to, fear of, and symptoms of anxious arousal. Examples of items are: 'It scares me when I feel faint', and 'Other people will notice when I feel shaky'. High scores on the Anxiety Sensitivity Index reflect a strong tendency to misinterpret arousal-related bodily sensations. Some other examples of self-rating instruments are: the Body Sensations Questionnaire, the Panic Attack Symptoms Questionnaire, the Panic Attack Cognitions Questionnaire, the Beck Anxiety Inventory, and the Spielberger State-Trait Anxiety Inventory.

Assessment for evaluating therapy

In a systematic approach, the patient will be assessed in some, or all, of the above ways at several points: before treatment begins, after a period of therapy, at the end of therapy, and at follow-up usually 6 and 12 months later. In this way the patient's progress can be measured formally and methodically.

The numerical scores, in particular, help to highlight the changes in the patient's feelings and behaviour. For example, assuming that therapy has been successful, a patient whose score on the Mobility Inventory was in the clinical range prior to treatment will have fallen to well within the normal range, e.g. from 75 to 40. Similarly, a person who started treatment with a significantly high Beck Depression Inventory score of 30, may have a score of less than 10 by the end of the treatment indicating an absence of depression.

Needless to say, even more important in evaluating the outcome of treatment are the frequency of panic episodes the patient experiences and their ratings of fear. If therapy is undertaken, the patient will be encouraged to maintain a simple daily record of panic episodes and other relevant events. Changes in avoidance behaviour, and the resumption of normal mobility, are second in importance only to the reduction or elimination of episodes of panic. Recording the non-occurrence of expected panics becomes increasingly important as therapy proceeds.

For those people who treat themselves, preferably after a professional assessment and advice, daily recordings and a regular completion of the key psychological questionnaires, are strongly advised.

Distinguishing between panic disorder and other disorders

As described in Chapter 1, many patients who suffer from any of the anxiety disorders have at least occasional episodes of panic. In some cases it is difficult to determine the interactions between the panics and the primary problem of the associated anxiety disorder. Not infrequently the interactions between the disorders shift during the course of therapy, and prior knowledge of the relation between the panics and the other disorder can be helpful.

In carrying out a full assessment of a panic disorder it is advisable to look into the presence of associated problems, including of course clinical depression (see p.72 above). Unless there is good reason fully to consider a co-morbid depression, the assessor may start with one or more psychometric screening tests, such as the widely used Beck Depression Scale, and follow it up, if the patient's score falls into the clinical range. The co-morbid presence of depression probably will determine the selection of treatment. For example, if it appears that the depression is disabling, it might be advisable to postpone psychological therapy until the patient has had an adequate course of anti-depressant medication.

Sometimes there is an overlap between obsessive–compulsive disorder and panic disorder, and it becomes necessary to assess whether or not the panics are secondary to, say, a fear of contamination. If so, the treatment plan may start with a reduction of this fear. Similarly, if the patient has co-morbid social phobia, it might be advisable to tackle the phobia first. If there is an associated problem of substance abuse, it might turn out that this problem is secondary to repeated episode of panic; it is not uncommon for sufferers from panic to 'self-medicate' with alcohol or drugs. In instances of co-morbid generalized anxiety disorder and panic, it may be necessary to tackle the two problems simultaneously.

Evidently it can be important to assess the psychological problems that are associated with the panic disorder, and a combination of systematic interviewing plus psychometric and behavioural tests is generally used. Patients who are obliged to run the gamut of assessments can became understandably bothered by the extensity and duration of the assessment, but in most cases it is necessary.

There are no laboratory tests for panic disorder.

9

Obstacles and complications

➲ Key Points

The obstacles to treatment by medications include negative attitudes to taking drugs, unpleasant side-effects, restrictions on diet, and cost.

The provision of comprehensive information about the particular medication is helpful and necessary; often it reduces misgivings about using the medication.

The provision of written material about the medication, including advice about precautions, is recommended.

In many instances the unpleasant side-effects diminish within a few weeks.

The major obstacle to psychological treatment is the limited availability of skilled clinical psychologists.

In the UK, the massive expansion of newly-trained psychologists will remove this obstacle and, as the programme is rolled out, waiting times should be sharply reduced.

Addition of the self-referral system will expedite psychological treatment.

If the person's panic disorder is associated with another significant psychological problem, such as depression, psychological treatment is more complicated and can be lengthy.

Important progress has been made in developing successful treatments for panic disorder, but some obstacles and complications are encountered.

Drug treatment

The main obstacles to pharmacological treatment are negative attitudes to medication, unpleasant side effects, and restrictions on diet.

As it is often necessary to take medication for long periods, the cost—to the patient or family, when the treatment is privately obtained, and to the clinic or hospital, when the treatment is provided by the health service—can be considerable. Negative attitudes to medication are not uncommon, and may be insuperable for those panic disorder patients who are frightened of any sensations that make them feel that they are losing control. For these patients psychological treatment is more appropriate.

As noted earlier, there are several side-effects of the drugs used to treat panics (see pp.41–44), and if severe or intrusive these may cause the patient to discontinue medication. Alternative drugs or lower doses may overcome this obstacle. It is highly desirable to prepare patients for possible side-effects and how they might be overcome, and the provision of written material about the medication is recommended. The provision of written and oral information about dietary or other restrictions, and possibly adverse reactions with other drugs, is always important. This is particularly so in the case of monoamine oxidase inhibitor drugs (MAOI).

The complications of drug treatment include interactions with other medications, unpleasant reactions when a drug is discontinued, and the possibility of relapse when the drugs are withdrawn. Relapses are particularly common with some benzodiazapine drugs, such as alprazolam, but this can sometimes be anticipated and modified by a gradual, tapered withdrawal over a period of up to three months.

Psychological treatment

The obstacles to psychological treatment are: the limited availability of clinical psychologists (which is currently being remedied by the programme to massively increase the number of psychological therapists), psychiatrists, and other specialist therapists, and negative or sceptical attitudes to such treatment. In addition, some outdated suspicions, embarrassment or fears about seeing a mental health professional, persist as an obstacle to such referrals. The recent introduction of a self-referral system to psychological services is likely to reduce the hesitation that some people feel about disclosing the nature of their panic problems. Once engaged in cognitive-behavioural therapy most patients find it acceptable, credible, and helpful. Complications can arise from coexisting problems. In many cases, the person is depressed as well as panicky, and this can interfere with treatment directly (due to lack of motivation, self-absorption, insomnia, lack of energy, or feelings of helplessness) or indirectly. Depressive thoughts and feelings may be tangled with the panic thoughts, and such confusion can impede progress. Marital or relationship problems can be a source of distress and confusion, obscuring the nature and the contributing causes of the panic disorder. Depending on the nature and seriousness of the coexisting problems, it may be necessary to deal with these before tackling the panics (such as reducing the depression), or arranging for the provision of marital counselling, where necessary. Patients who are substance abusers can present special problems; for example, the progress of treatment of a patient with panic disorder and agoraphobia was impeded by intermittent bouts of excessive drinking that left him shaky and highly anxious.

When the panic disorder is associated with severe agoraphobia, the patient may find it extremely difficult to travel to treatment. Energetic attempts need to be made, directly or via friends/relatives or family doctor, to encourage the patient to attend, even if they have to be accompanied in the early stages. In the most severe, housebound, cases it may be necessary to begin the treatment in the patient's home. Such domiciliary work is extremely time-consuming, and may not be available from all clinics. Self-help treatment manuals and treatment advice by regular telephone contact are increasingly used by services, with some success.

Physical illnesses

If the panic disorder patient also has a significant physical illness, such as a cardiovascular disorder or hypoglycaemia, this may complicate treatment. Some of the anti-panic drugs may interact adversely with the patient's other medications and are to be avoided. Some illnesses can also complicate psychological treatment. For example, the patient's dizziness may be a symptom of some disorder of the ear and not a manifestation of anxiety. Similarly, treatment of a panic patient who really does have a cardiac problem can be complicated. In these cases, the therapist will work closely with the family doctor or cardiologist. In a small but significant minority of cases, investigation for possible physical illness is crucial.

10

Some practical advice

➜ Key Points

* For people who are concerned about intense feelings of anxiety, a list of preliminary questions can provide a starting point for considering the possibility of a panic disorder.

* The list of questions set out below can also provide some preliminary assistance in sorting out the possibility that a relative or friend might be struggling with a panic disorder.

* Suggestions are made about how to seek help.

* The initial assessment of the problem will include interviews, questionnaires and tests; with permission, the person's relatives and friends may be consulted.

* An outline of the planning and conduct of treatment is provided.

* Suggestions are made about how the affected person can facilitate treatment.

* Advice about self-treatment is provided.

* Advice is provided about how to consolidate progress after the completion of treatment.

Is there a problem?

We all experience anxiety at one time or another, and a significant minority of the population experience occasional episodes of panic. Most people are rarely concerned or worried about the occasional episode of panic, particularly if the cause of the panic is easily recognized and understandable, such as a near collision while driving. However, repeated episodes of severe panic, particularly those that come 'out of the blue', are distressing and troubling. They very often are associated with or a direct cause of significant anxiety about one's health. If you have high, continuing levels of anxiety and repeated episodes of panic, if your panics interfere with your personal life, work, leisure activities, and find it necessary to restrict your movements, then you should consider seeking help.

Some key questions

At this stage it is helpful to ask yourself some questions about the problem:

- Are you having recurrent episodes of intense fear (panics) which arise rapidly and last for ten minutes or more?
- During a panic do ever feel that your life is threatened?
- During a panic do you ever feel a sense of impending doom?
- Are any of these episodes totally unexpected?
- Are these episodes of panic a source of considerable distress and concern?
- Do you tend to worry about them for weeks or months after they occur?
- Have the panics generated serious anxiety about your health?
- Do you find yourself constantly avoiding certain activities, places, or people as a result of the panics?
- Have your job, social life, recreation, become more difficult as a result of the panics?
- Are your panics a source of significant embarrassment for you?
- Are your panics a significant nuisance or hindrance to other people?
- Do you find yourself spending a great deal of time worrying about the episodes of panic and their possible meaning for your health?

If your answer to at least some of these questions is 'yes', then your anxiety and panic probably do require attention and you may wish to consider taking action.

Concern about a member of the family or a friend

The same considerations arise when a spouse, relative, or friend observes a high level of anxiety, panic, and increasing avoidance behaviour in another person. If the affected person shows major changes in behaviour, and is becoming increasingly dependent on friends and relatives to get out to do the shopping or to travel to work, then the family may be justifiably worried. As mentioned earlier, daily or weekly fluctuations in the affected person's level of anxiety, tendency to have panics, and immobility, can be a source of puzzlement in the family. If persistent difficulties are observed despite the fluctuations, the family needs to be concerned.

In some cases, the affected person attempts to conceal the true nature of the problem. In one example, a young married woman concealed the fact that she was having panics and was, therefore, frightened of going out on her own. She tried to ensure that she was always accompanied when she went out of the house. When this was not possible, she would excuse herself and simply stay home ('I couldn't go shopping today because I had a headache'). Eventually it emerged that, unbeknown to her husband, she had been the victim of an attempted sexual attempt a few years earlier and had developed a fear of travelling alone. When her avoidance of going out unaccompanied became evident to the husband, he encouraged her to seek professional help. She was much improved by a course of psychological therapy.

Seeking help

Once it is recognized that there is a problem, the best course of action is to seek professional advice. In some cases it may be possible to deal with the difficulties without much professional assistance, but in most cases seeking the advice of a qualified professional, at least in order to obtain a full assessment, is a sensible first step.

Finding a therapist

With the recent introduction of self-referral psychological services, it is possible to get assistance directly. Many people might prefer to visit their family doctor in the first instance. As described previously, your family doctor is in a position to provide useful information and reassurance, and may decide to provide psychological or pharmacological treatment. If the problem is particularly severe or complex, or if you fail to derive significant benefit from the initial treatment, your doctor may then consider a referral to a specialist, usually a clinical psychologist or a psychiatrist.

Your local health service should be able to direct your doctor to a suitable therapeutic service. You can also obtain useful information from the NHS Websites. The British Association for Behavioural and Cognitive Psychotherapies (BABCP) can advise on therapists in each area. Most of the therapists work within the National Health Service in Britain, but if you prefer to see someone privately, the BABCP will be able to advise you. General advice on the services of clinical psychologists and psychiatrists can be obtained from their respective professional organizations, the British Psychological Society and the Royal College of Psychiatrists. Advice is also obtainable from MIND, the National Association for Mental Health, and from various self-help organizations such as Phobic Action, No Panic, and First Steps to Freedom.

In the United States, healthcare provisions vary considerably from state to state, but most are well-supplied with psychiatrists and clinical psychologists. Information about clinical psychologists who specialize in providing cognitive-behaviour therapy can be obtained from the American Psychological Association and from the Association for the Advancement of Behavior and Cognitive Therapy. In addition, a voluntary non-profit organization called the Anxiety Disorders Association of America, provides useful information and advice about the disorder. The National Institute of Mental Health is also a useful resource.

In Canada, the clinical services vary from province to province, as do the healthcare insurance policies. In some provinces, psychological therapy is included as part of the comprehensive insurance policy but in others, such as British Columbia, it is not. However, psychological treatment can be obtained at subsidized rates, or free, at some hospitals or university-associated clinics. Information about such services is usually available from the Psychological Association of each province or from the Canadian Psychological Association. Advice about psychiatric care can be obtained from the Canadian Psychiatric Association and from the provincial psychiatric associations. The Canadian Mental Health Association will also provide advice and information.

In Australia, the Australian Psychological Society and the Royal Australian and New Zealand College of Psychiatrists are the main professional organizations that can provide information about services. Psychological treatment services in Australia are of a high standard and treatment is subsidized.

Addresses of the organizations mentioned above, and of a few other useful centres and agencies, are given in Appendix 4.

The therapist's assessment

When you go for your assessment, the therapist will try to collect as much relevant information as possible, and it may well take more than a single interview to complete the full assessment. The therapist is likely to request information described in the previous chapters. The therapist is also likely to ask you to complete some questionnaires, inventories, checklists, or other short tests. If your problem includes a significant amount of avoidance behaviour, these will probably be supplemented by a behavioural avoidance test, in which you will be asked to travel various distances while observed by the therapist (such as walk from the clinic entrance to the shops two blocks away). The therapist may ask you to keep a diary and record of your anxiety and/or panics as they occur in the week or two following the initial assessment, like the ones shown in Figures 8.1 and 8.2.

The therapist may wish to discuss the problem with a family member or close friend, subject to your agreement. If you are severely agoraphobic, verging on being housebound, it sometimes is necessary for the therapist to include a home visit as part of the assessment.

The planning and conduct of psychological therapy

In planning the treatment programme, your therapist will discuss with you the two main elements of treatment: the cognitive analysis and the behavioural exposure exercises. Nowadays, virtually all treatment of panic disorders is carried out on an outpatient basis, and hospitalization is rarely considered to be an option. Indeed, it is only in the most exceptional or complicated cases that admission to a hospital would be considered; even then it is likely to be for a short period.

Throughout the therapy you are likely to be asked to keep regular records of your daily levels of anxiety, and the occurrence or non-occurrence of episodes of panic. You may also be asked to keep records of the strength of some of your panic-related beliefs (such as, 'I have panics because I have a weak heart'). The occurrence of particular stresses or unusual events should also be recorded. These recordings of your progress are important, as they provide a good deal of continuous information, and the progress and modification of treatment is dependent largely on the completeness and accuracy of the information that is coming in. Relying on your recollection of various events that have taken place over a two- or four-week period is not a substitute for the daily recording of events as they occur. The records also serve a useful function in helping you to plot your progress, which is usually gradual and steady, and which in turn acts as a source of inspiration and encouragement for further efforts.

In some cases it might be necessary to have the active involvement of a relative or friend in the planning and conduct of the exposure exercises. However, in order to avoid any ambiguity that might lead to conflict within the family, the role that the relative plays should be clearly defined and detailed, with specific instructions and guidance provided by the therapist. It is also advisable for the relatives and friends to remember that the early progress that the patient makes is not a sign that the problem is entirely solved. Sometimes relatives and friends expect unrealistically rapid progress and put unnecessary and unhelpful pressure on the patient. They should also be aware of the fluctuations in fear, panic, and avoidance referred to earlier, and that these fluctuations may persist for a time during the conduct of the therapy.

What you can do to facilitate the treatment

Psychological therapy for panic disorder is a joint venture. The therapist can do very little without your active co-operation, because a large part of the treatment will depend upon your effort. To some extent the role of the therapist merges with that of an instructor or tutor, in which you are given advice and direction in order to carry out the cognitive and behavioural changes that are necessary.

Both the cognitive and behavioural work can be distressing and difficult at times, and in the early stages might provoke uneasiness and fear. But if you are strongly motivated to overcome the problem, you will find that with the help of the therapist, you can endure and persist until the problem is successfully dealt with. Occasional returns of anxiety, or even the occasional episode of panic, should not be seen as a failure, and you should not allow yourself to be discouraged by them. Your improvement should be progressive and smooth, but do not be too surprised if there are some disappointments and some difficult days or even weeks. The beneficial effects are of lasting value in most cases.

As you gradually improve during the course of treatment you may well find that you have to readjust your behaviour. If you have been immobilized, partly or largely, by your panics and their consequences, you will need to re-establish your old ways of travel and mobility, and revive the social and other contacts that had lapsed because of your difficulties. Members of your family will also have to make adjustments and get used to the significant alterations in your behaviour. For example, they may need quite a few reminders before they recognize that they no longer have to accompany you on shopping expeditions, or ensure that someone is always in the house when you are at home. Your increasing independence will have major effects on the lives of your family members, and on their relationship with you. The family of one patient, who had been severely affected by panic disorder and related restrictions in mobility and who improved considerably after treatment, said, 'Our life has completely changed. We live normally once again'.

After therapy

When you have achieved significant improvement, do not expect to be totally free of anxiety. It often happens that the episodes of panic decrease or stop altogether, and the frightening thoughts that accompany them also wane. However, some of the thoughts may linger on in a milder fashion at the back of your mind, and you may feel that you are not absolutely free of them. Try to remember that anxiety is a universal experience, and that a very occasional episode of panic need not signify the return of a significant problem. Many people have occasional episodes of panic but continue to live a perfectly normal and full life.

Once successfully treated, the chances of a major relapse are not very high. There may, however, be occasional lapses in which you sense a return of the urge to avoid situations formerly associated with panic. You should try to resist the return of avoidance behaviour, even if it is difficult to do so at the time, because it can become the source of a return of fear. In fact, it is best to regard the return of even mild urges to avoid as a sure sign that you need to re-introduce some of the exposure exercises that you originally completed during treatment (keep on using public transport, do your shopping regularly, do your physical exercises regularly). You can 'immunize' yourself by carrying out some of the exposure exercises on a regular basis, just as an athlete has to continue practising regularly even when no events are imminent. Keeping active and psychologically fit is the best way of giving yourself protection against the return of the problem.

If, however, you do experience more than one severe episode of panic, you should return to the therapist for further advice, and possibly a few booster treatments. These tend to be highly effective, and it is unusual for a successfully treated patient to require a second full course of treatment. Many therapists ask their patients to return after several months, anyway, in order to check on progress and arrange for booster sessions, if necessary.

Self-treatment

If your problem is not very severe, and if there are no other complications, it might be possible to complete the treatment without professional assistance.

If you have other psychological problems, especially depression, it is unwise to attempt a course of self-treatment, and you would do well to seek professional advice early on. If you habitually use a good deal of alcohol or drugs, such as benzodiazepines, self-help should not be attempted without first consulting your doctor. Or, if the episodes of panic are associated with distressing and troubling thoughts about your health, or even your life, then the assistance of a professional should be sought. The problem that lends itself most directly to self-treatment is avoidance. If you have few panic episodes *and* mild agoraphobia without any complications, then you might be a good candidate for a self-treatment approach. You should select a small number of clearly defined behavioural targets that you wish to achieve, such as: walk to the local post office and back, walk around the block at a quiet time, go to the nearest supermarket for a short time, and so on. It is sensible to start with a fairly easy goal initially and then, as you begin to make progress walking or driving towards the goal, become more ambitious and expand your targets to include more distant and more difficult targets. It is advisable to carry out these self-exposure exercises on a regular basis, otherwise you run the risk of losing some of the benefits during the long intervals in-between. The complete discontinuation of such exercises is unwise, as you might become 'rusty' and allow your confidence to fade.

It is sometimes helpful to have a relative or friend monitor your progress and plan the next targets on your list. Whether you work entirely on your own, or with the assistance of a friend or relative, you will find it helpful to keep good records of your progress. They will make it easier for you to plan your targets and to identify any difficulties that may arise; you can use a form similar to the one that is shown in Figures 10.1 and 10.2.

Date:	
Target:	
Time:	
Alone or accompanied:	
If accompanied, by whom:	
Anxiety (0–100)	
	Before:
	During (highest):
	After:
Any panics:	
Comments:	

Figure 10.1 A blank example of a record sheet for an exposure session.

Date:	7th May
Target:	Buy something in supermarket
Time:	3 p.m.
Alone or accompanied:	Accompanied
If accompanied, by whom:	Bob (my husband)
Anxiety (0–100)	

	Before:	30
	During (highest):	70
	After:	20

Any panics:	None	
Comments:	Felt quite anxious going in, as it was very crowded. Held Bob's hand when we entered. Picked up a few things quickly, it wasn't too bad then. Felt anxious again while waiting to pay at the check-out. Having Bob near me helped. He kept talking to me. Felt good when we came out.	

Figure 10.2 A completed example of a record sheet for an exposure session.

If you tend to be generally anxious, or you find that you are getting exceedingly anxious during the exercises, a useful addition to your self-treatment programme is training in relaxation and breathing retraining. A brief guide to these methods is provided in Appendix 3. You should attempt to find the time to practise regularly. You can use the relaxation and breathing exercises before you set out on an exposure exercise, during the exercise if you begin to feel tense or anxious, and as a way of reducing anxiety and tension at other times.

A number of sound self-help books and tapes are now available. They provide information about the disorder, and also give structured, graded steps that can be used in self-treatment. You may find such resources quite useful in treating yourself. Some of these are listed in Appendix 5.

Some organizations that provide information and advice about treatment are listed in Appendix 4.

A word of caution

A word of caution is needed about self-treatment. It is not advisable to undertake treatment entirely on your own unless your problems are relatively straightforward and consist mainly of avoidance behaviour. Even if you carry out much or most of the therapy entirely by yourself, it is often useful to discuss your problems at the outset with a qualified therapist. The therapist will be able to advise you about whether or not a self-therapy programme is suitable and likely to be effective, and may also agree to monitor your progress from time to time. For people who do not have easy access to a therapist, a self-treatment programme may be the only option, but even here, an initial assessment and some form of monitoring, even by telephone, is advisable.

A word of hope

Remember that episodes of panic are experienced by many people, and are not a sign of something sinister. Panic disorder, even when it is quite severe and handicapping, is a treatable condition. With the right advice, appropriate therapy, and your own effort, it can be overcome. Many, many people have done so.

11

Common questions

What is the effect of repeated episodes of panic on my long-term health?

Many patients worry that the effects of their episodes of panic may be cumulative, as in: 'Can my body stand the repeated stress?'. The recurrent panics are distressing and accompanied by unpleasant bodily sensations but there is no evidence that they damage one's health. The damage, if any, tends to be psychological and generates anxiety, adverse changes in one's activities, restrictions on mobility, and a loss of self-confidence.

Does panic disorder develop into major mental illness?

No. In many cases panic disorder is associated with other types of anxiety, such as social phobia, agoraphobia, and/or depression, but it is not associated with major mental illnesses.

Is panic disorder a mental illness?

Panic disorder is a psychological problem and is not related to schizophrenia, mania, or any other major mental illness. People who experience recurrent episodes of panic are not insane and nor are they going to go insane. Panic disorder is a problem of anxiety, and has nothing to do with insanity as that term is broadly used.

Do people ever die from panic?

No. Panics are distressing very unpleasant experiences, but invariably come to an end; they are self-limiting. Most episodes of panic last between 10 and 20 minutes, and tend to leave the person shaken and tired.

How likely is it that I will lose control during an episode of panic and do something bizarre, harmful, or dangerous?

A fear of losing control is common during episodes of panic, but bizarre or dangerous actions rarely occur.

During a panic I feel that it will never end; do panics ever last for days on end, or even longer?

Distressing panics may seem to last forever but, as mentioned above, the average duration of an episode is from 10 to 20 minutes. They are self-limiting and the unpleasant physical sensations subside spontaneously, if gradually. After experiencing an episode of panic the person tends to feel shaken and drained, and often will be left with a residue of some anxiety.

Will my children inherit panic disorder?

Panic disorder, as such, is not inherited; there is, however, evidence of the inheritance of a predisposition to experience excessive anxiety, which is probably more common among relatives of people with panic disorder. A predisposition does not mean that someone will necessarily develop the disorder in question. As a group, the first-degree relatives (parents, children, brothers, sisters) of a person with panic disorder are more likely than the average to experience a similar disorder at some time in their lives. These are, however, group averages and it is not possible to predict exactly who will and who will not experience problems.

Should I conceal the fact that I have panic disorder?

There is no good reason to conceal it, and certainly no reason for embarrassment or shame. It remains true that there is lot of ignorance about panic disorder and other psychological problems, despite some useful advances in public education, and ill-informed people may misunderstand the nature of your difficulties. The decision to enlighten them rests with you. Close friends and relatives tend to be more sympathetic and understanding, and in almost all instances it is best to speak openly about your anxiety and the associated problems. You certainly should feel free to discuss your feelings fully with your doctor.

In some circumstances, ill-advised employers may be prejudiced against a person with a panic disorder, and this is one of the few times, perhaps the only one, in which discretion may be needed.

If you wish to speak about your panic disorder outside of therapy, and also wish to listen to the experiences of other people, you may do well to join one of the many self-help groups that have been formed over the past few years.

Some useful addresses are provided in Appendix 4. If there is no such organization in your area, you may even consider starting one.

Will my children start to imitate my panics?

This is extremely unlikely. Depending on age, your children will be aware of days and times when you appear to be tense and/or anxious. If your symptoms are severe and frequent they are likely to be concerned about you and may even acquire anxiety themselves. However, it is improbable that they will display episodes of panic, even if they observe you experiencing panics on occasion.

What is the long-term outlook for panic disorder?

At present we have insufficient information about the natural (i.e. untreated) course of panic disorder, but in agoraphobia, up to one-third of all people experience some spontaneous improvement within two years of the onset of the problem. Descriptions given by panic disorder patients suggest that the course of the untreated disorder is a fluctuating one in many cases. But these accounts are retrospective, and may be inaccurate. The main reason for our ignorance about the untreated course of panic disorder is that the problem is now readily diagnosed, and effective treatments are available. On current evidence, which is sparse but accumulating, the long-term outlook after successful cognitive-behavioural therapy is highly favourable. Comparatively few relapses occur.

Even after successful treatment, however, a recurrence of stress, the onset of depression, or suffering a traumatic event, can result in a partial return of the problem. In these cases, a short course of booster treatments may be required.

With some of the medications, notably benzodiazepines, relapse can be a major problem when the drugs are stopped. In order to reduce the prospect of a relapse, the medication should be tapered off very gradually, under medical supervision.

How can I find out about and reduce side-effects of medications?

Most medications that produce beneficial therapeutic effects are also prone to produce some unwanted side-effects. The most common side-effects for the main anti-panic medications are set out on pp.41–44. There are also authoritative internet websites that provide details of most medications. There are wide individual differences in the occurrence of side-effects, and it is difficult to predict exactly what to expect for each patient; some patients can tolerate one type of medication but react badly to another. As a result, the search for the correct medication and the most effective, tolerable dose for a particular patient, may require patience. Your doctor will discuss in advance the possible side-effects of your medication with you, and you must keep the doctor in the picture about the side-effects that you experience. Fortunately, most patients find that they gradually become accustomed to the side-effects and worry less about them as the benefits of treatment become evident.

Will I be on medication for the rest of my life?

No. After a prolonged period free, or almost free, of panic episodes and of lowered anxiety, you can discuss with your doctor the viability/timing of coming off the drugs. Depending on the severity and duration of the original problem, a panic-free period of 3–12 months is a rough guide for reviewing the role of the medications. Two problems can arise when medications are phased out. If the withdrawal of the medication is too abrupt, unpleasant effects may be experienced—nausea, tension, irritability, insomnia—the so-called 'discontinuation effect'. There is also a risk that when people who have been taking a particular drug for a long period stop abruptly, they might have a temporary rebound of the original symptoms. Both of these unpleasant reactions can be avoided by a gradual tapering-off of the medication. A second problem is relapse after stopping the medication. Relapses are common when certain drugs are withdrawn, notably benzodiazepines, but not usual with other drugs. You and your doctor might decide to re-start the same medication or switch to another type.

Can hypnosis cure panic attacks?

Claims are often made by various people that hypnosis can 'cure' episodes of panic quickly. In hypnotherapy, the person is brought to a trance-like state by suggestion, and in this state, they may be told that there will be no more panic attacks. Unfortunately, such post-hypnotic suggestions do not produce lasting beneficial effects. The main problem with hypnosis, and other alternative therapies, is that they have not been properly evaluated, and what little evaluation has been done has not produced satisfactory evidence of efficacy. This is in contrast to the treatments described in Chapters 6 and 7, which have been the subject of systematic research that meets professional standards.

Can I learn to treat myself?

If your disorder is uncomplicated you may well be able to help yourself by following one of the self-help programmes now available, or following the suggestions given in this book. It is, however, worthwhile considering an assessment by a therapist or clinician before embarking on a self-help programme, and also checking in when you have completed the programme. Additionally, you may wish to obtain advice, support, and encouragement from a self-help group or a self-help organization.

Is it true that drinking coffee can cause panic attacks?

Caffeine, which is present in many common drinks such as coffee, tea, cola, and cocoa, does not cause panic disorder, but it can exacerbate panic symptoms. Caffeine has also been used in laboratory studies to induce panic attacks in patients with panic disorder. Many patients suffering from panic disorder learn to avoid caffeine, through experience. This does not mean that drinking coffee, or other beverages that contain caffeine, in moderation causes panic symptoms.

I have been advised by friends to take some herbal preparations for my panics. Will these help?

Many people use herbal preparations for a variety of psychological problems, and there are those who prefer natural substances to psychiatric drugs, which are not universally popular. Some people claim that certain herbal preparations have a calming effect and help to reduce their panic episodes. However, there have been few systematic evaluations of the effectiveness of these products. One must also be aware of possible adverse reactions when taking herbal products while on prescribed medication.

Do people who suffer from episodes of panic feel frightened all the time?

No, they do not. When they are not threatened by the prospect of a panic, or threatened by the prospect of a situation that might evoke a reaction associated with panics, they engage in ordinary, normal activities.

Is a person who experiences episodes of panic incapable of ever performing courageously?

People who suffer from panic disorder are capable of performing courageously in situations that demand courage, but which have no connection to those situations that are associated with past episodes of panic. For example, most patients who have difficult, dangerous jobs, such as policemen, fire-fighters, soldiers, can continue performing their work, even while receiving treatment for a panic disorder. In addition, patients with panic disorder usually perform satisfactorily in emergency situations, e.g. motor vehicle accidents. If, however, a person who has a difficult, dangerous job develops a panic disorder that impinges directly on his work, it might be necessary to arrange for disability leave in order to obtain treatment.

Appendix 1

The mobility inventory

Please indicate the degree to which you avoid the following places or situations because of discomfort or anxiety. Rate your amount of avoidance when you are with a trusted companion and when you are alone. Do this by using the following scale.

1 = Never avoid
2 = Rarely avoid
3 = Avoid about half the time
4 = Avoid most of the time
5 = Always avoid

(You may use numbers halfway between those listed when you think it is appropriate, e.g. 3½ or 4½). Write your score in the blanks for each situation or place under both conditions: when accompanied, and, when alone. Leave blank those situations that do not apply to you.

Places	When accompanied	When alone
Theatres	——	——
Supermarkets	——	——
Classrooms	——	——
Department stores	——	——
Restaurants	——	——
Museums	——	——
Elevators	——	——
Auditoriums or stadiums	——	——
Parking garages	——	——
High places		
Tell how high	——	——
Enclosed spaces (e.g. tunnels)	——	——

Open spaces

    (A) Outside (e.g. fields, wide   ——   ——
         streets, courtyards)

    (B) Inside (e.g. large rooms,   ——   ——
         lobbies)

Riding in

Buses   ——   ——

Trains   ——   ——

Subways   ——   ——

Airplanes   ——   ——

Boats   ——   ——

Driving or riding in car

    (A) At any time   ——   ——

    (B) On motorways   ——   ——

Situations

Standing in lines   ——   ——

Crossing bridges   ——   ——

Parties or social gatherings   ——   ——

Walking on the street   ——   ——

Staying at home alone   NA   ——

Being far away from home   ——   ——

Other (specify)   ——   ——

We define a panic as:

(1) a high level of anxiety accompanied by

(2) strong body reactions (heart palpitations, sweating, muscle tremors, dizziness, nausea) with

(3) the temporary loss of the ability to plan, think, or reason and

(4) an intense desire to escape or flee the situation.

(Note: this is different from high anxiety or fear alone.)

Please indicate the total number of panic attacks you have had in the last 7 days   ——

Appendix 2

The cognitions questionnaire

Below are some thoughts or ideas that may pass through your mind when you are nervous or frightened.

Please indicate how often each thought occurs when you are nervous. Rate from 1 to 5 using the scale below:

1 = Thought never occurs.
2 = Thought rarely occurs.
3 = Thought occurs during half of the times I am nervous.
4 = Thought usually occurs.
5 = Thought always occurs when I am nervous.

Thought	Rating
I am going to be sick	——
I am going to faint	——
I must have a brain tumour	——
I shall have a heart-attack	——
I shall choke to death	——
I am going to act foolishly	——
I am going blind	——
I shall not be able to control myself	——
I shall hurt someone	——
I am going to have a stroke	——
I am going to go insane	——
I am going to scream	——

I am going to babble or talk in a funny way   ——

I shall be paralyzed by fear   ——

OTHER IDEAS NOT LISTED (PLEASE DESCRIBE AND RATE THEM)

     ——

     ——

From Chambless *et al.* (1984). See Appendix 5 for full reference.
Reproduced with permission.

Appendix 3

Learning to relax: a simple guide

Do your relaxation exercises in a quiet room, at a time when you are not likely to be disturbed. Sit comfortably in an armchair. Make sure that your clothes are not tight. Remove belts, spectacles, and shoes.

Learn to relax by first tensing and then relaxing various muscle groups of the body, one at a time. Keep eyes closed throughout. At each step, keep the muscles tensed, quite hard, for 6–8 seconds, and notice the tension. Concentrate on the muscles, and notice the tension. Then relax the muscles, and keep them relaxed for 45–50 seconds. Again, concentrate on the muscles, and notice how the feelings of relaxation differ from those of tension. You can learn to time yourself quite easily by slowly counting for the first few times. Remember to repeat the tense–relax cycle for each muscle group before you move on to the next. When you tense a group of muscles, take a breath and hold it until you relax the muscles, and release the breath slowly as you relax.

The order in which to tense and relax the various muscle groups is given below. For each muscle group, a strategy for making them tense is given. For some, alternative strategies are suggested. Before you actually start the proper relaxation exercises, learn the way in which each muscle group can be effectively tensed. Try out one at a time, and master it. Where alternatives are suggested, decide which one is going to be your regular strategy.

Once this is done, you can begin the actual sessions.

1. *Right hand and forearm*: Tense the muscles by making a tight fist; or, try pressing the inner part of the finger tips against the base of the thumb. Relax by slowly opening the hand.
2. *Right biceps*: Tense muscles by pushing your elbow into the arm of the chair, or by pressing the elbow and the upper arm into the side of the rib cage. Relax by returning to original position.
3. *Left hand and forearm*: As for the right hand and forearm.
4. *Left biceps*: As for right biceps.
(*Note*: If you are left-handed, do steps 3 and 4 first, followed by steps 1 and 2.)

5. *Forehead*: Tense by raising your eyebrows as high as possible with your eyes still closed. Relax by returning eyebrows to normal position.

6. *Upper cheeks and nose*: Tense by squinting and screwing up your eyes, and wrinkling your nose. Relax by returning to normal position.

7. *Lower cheeks and jaws*: Tense by clenching your teeth together and pulling back the corners of your mouth. Relax by unclenching the teeth and bringing mouth back to normal.

8. *Neck*: Tense by pulling your chin into your chest, but not quite touching it. Relax by returning to original position.

9. *Shoulder and chest*: Tense by raising and pulling your shoulder blades towards each other. Relax by returning to original position.

10. *Stomach and abdomen*: Tense by pulling in your abdomen as much as you can. You can also tense these muscles by pushing out your stomach and abdomen. Relax by returning to original state.

11. *Right leg*: Tense by straightening the whole leg from the hip, parallel to the floor. Relax by lowering and resting the leg on the floor again.

12. *Right foot*: Tense by pushing your heel into the floor and curling your toes upwards, i.e. towards you. Relax by returning to original position.

13. *Left leg*: As for the right leg.

14. *Left foot*: As for the right foot.

(*Note*: If your dominant leg is the left one, do steps 13 and 14 before 11 and 12.)

15. *Whole body*: Tense as many of the muscle groups as you can all at once, making yourself into a 'ball of tension'. You will find that you can tense most of the muscle groups together; in fact, if you use the tension strategies suggested above, there will be only two of these items that you will not be able to do while doing everything else. One is the raising of the eyebrows, but the eyebrows can be tensed by wrinkling them when you screw up the eyes. The second is the pushing of your heels into the floor, but with your legs stretched, you will still be able to curl your toes up towards you.

Remember that each step is to be done twice, including the last 'all-body' step. Remember also to take a breath and hold it when the muscles are kept tense, and to release the breath as you relax the muscles.

After the whole sequence is completed, continue to sit in a relaxed state for several minutes. At this point, you may imagine a pleasant scene, like a peaceful beach or a flower garden. With practice, when you become more skilled in relaxing yourself, you will find the exercises become quite easy. After some weeks of practice, you will be able to relax yourself by simply tensing and relaxing the entire body, i.e. the last step of the sequence given above, without going through the separate steps. With even more practice, many people acquire the ability to relax very effectively simply by concentrating on making their muscles relaxed without having first to tense them.

If you wish to do your relaxation exercises lying down on a bed or the floor, only minor changes to the above programme are needed. For each leg, what you will need to do is to raise it from the bed or floor to form an angle of about 30 degrees. Relax by lowering and resting the leg on the bed or floor.

There is no particular time of the day when relaxation should be practised, but avoid doing it when you are very sleepy, to avoid falling asleep while relaxing. Try to do it daily in the early stages, so you will quickly become good at it.

There are different sequences of muscle groups suggested by different authors for relaxation exercises. There is no particular advantage of one over the others. What is important is to use a sequence that is fairly logical, as the one given here, not a random or haphazard one. You should use the same sequence regularly, so it will be easier to learn and master it.

There are cassette tapes available commercially, which give recorded instructions for relaxation training. Using one of these can be useful in the early stages, but it is important to wean yourself gradually away from the cassette, as the aim is to learn to relax without any external aid. The following are some good cassettes that are commercially available:

Relax and enjoy it, by Robert Sharpe, available from Aleph One Ltd, The Old Courthouse, High Street, Bottisham, Cambridge CB5 9BA.

Self-help relaxation, by Jane Madders, available from Relaxation for Living Ltd, 29 Burwood Park Road, Walton-on-Thames, Surrey KT12 5LH.

How to relax, by Rachel Norris & Christina Kuchemann, which comes with *Managing anxiety: a user's manual*, by Helen Kennerley, available from the Psychology Department, Warneford Hospital, Oxford OX3 7JX.

The *relaxation cassette*, by Reinhard Kowalski, available from Winslow Press, Telford Road, Bicester OX6 OTS.

The relaxation tapes (and videos) produced by First Steps to Freedom, 7 Avon Court, School Lane, Kenilworth, Warwickshire CV8 2GX.

Appendix 4

Useful organizations

British Association for Behavioural and Cognitive Psychotherapies
Globe Centre
PO Box 9
Accrington
BB5 2DG
www.bahcp.org.uk

British Psychological Society
St Andrews House
48 Princess Road East
Leicester LEI 7DR
www.bps.org.uk

Royal College of Psychiatrists
17 Belgrave Square
London SW1X 8PG
www.rcpsych.ac.uk

MIND, National Association for Mental Health
22 Harley Street
London W1N 2ED
www.mind.org.uk

First Steps to Freedom
7 Avon Court
Kenilworth
Warwickshire CV8 2GX

National Phobic Society
Zion Community Resource Centre
339 Stretford Road
Manchester M15 42Y

No Panic
93 Brands Farm Way
Randlay
Telford TF3 2JQ
www.no-panic.co.uk

Association for Advancement of Behavior Therapy
305 Seventh Avenue
16th Floor
New York, NY 10001
www.aabt.org

American Psychiatric Association
1000 Wilson Boulevard
Suite 1825
Arlington
VA 22209 – 3901

American Psychological Association
750 First Street, NE
Washington, DC 20002 – 4242
www.apa.org

Anxiety Disorders Association of America

8730 Georgia Avenue

Suite 600

Silver Spring, MD 20910

www.adaa.org

National Institute of Mental Health (NIMH)

Office of Communications

6001 Executive Boulevard

Room 8184

MSC 9663

Berhesda, MD 20892 – 9663

www.nimh.nih.gov

CANADA

Canadian Psychiatric Association

Suite 200

237 Argyle Avenue

Ottawa

Ontario

K2P 1B8

cpa@cpa-apc.org

Canadian Psychological Association

151 Slater Street

Suite 205

Ottawa

Ontario K1P 5H3

Canadian Mental Health Association

8 King Street East

Suite 810

Toronto

Ontario M5C 1B5

www.cmha.ca

Anxiety Disorders Association, British Columbia (ADABC)

4438 West 10th Avenue

Suite 119

Vancouver

British Columbia V6R 4R8

www.anxietybc.com

AUSTRALIA

Australian Psychological Society

PO Box 38

Flinders Lane Post Office

Melbourne

VIC 8009

www.psychsociety.com.au

Royal Australian and New Zealand College of Psychiatrists

309 La Trobe Street

Melbourne

VIC 3000

www.ranzcp.org

Australian Association for Cognitive and Behaviour Therapy

www.aacbt.org

Mental Health Association NSW Inc.

ada@mentalhealth.asn.au

CRUFAD (Clinical Research Unit for Anxiety and Depression)

St Vincent's Hospital

299 Forbes Street

Darlington, Sydney

NSCO 2010

www. crufad. org

www.crufad.com

Appendix 5

Further reading

The NICE Report on Panic Disorders and Generalized Anxiety Disorders, in an abridged form:

www.nice.org.uk/CG022quickrefguide

Technical

There are several major books that cover the topic of panic disorder. These include:

Barlow, D.H. (2002) *Anxiety and its disorders*, 2nd edn. Guilford Press, New York, USA.

An outstanding book on the whole range of anxiety disorders.

Barlow, D.H. and Craske, M.G. (1988) The phenomenology of panic. In: *Panic: pyscholoigcal perspectives* (eds S. Rachman and J.D. Maser), pp. 11–35, Lawrence Erlbaum, Hillsdale, NJ, USA.

Chambless, D.L., Caputo, G.C., Bright, P., and Gallagher, R. (1984) Assessment of fear in agarophobics: the Body Sensations Questionnaire and the Agoraphobic Cognitions Questionnaire. *Journal of Coculting and Clinical Psychology*, **52**, 1090–7.

Chambless, D.L., Caputo, G.C., Jasin, S.E., Gracely, E.J., and Williams (1985) The Mobility Inventory for agoraphobia. *Behaviour Research and Therapy*, **23**, 35–44.

Clark, D.M. (1986). A cognitive approach to panic. *Behaviour Research and Therapy*, **23**, 35–44.

Clark, D.M. (1999) Anxiety disorders: why they persist and how to treat them. *Behaviour Research and Therapy*, **37**, Supplement, pp. S5–S27.

A thorough and critical analysis of all aspects of panic disorder.

Craske, M.G. (1999) *Anxiety disorders*. Westview Press, Boulder, Colorado, USA.

An excellent, comprehensive account and analysis of all the anxiety disorders.

Rachman, S. (2004) *Anxiety*, 2nd edn. Psychology Press, Hove.

Includes an analysis of the debate on the nature of panic disorder.

Wolfe, B.E. and Maser, J.D. (eds) (1994) *Treatment of panic disorder*. American Psychiatric Press, Washington DC, USA.

This book, which reports the proceedings of a major Consensus Development Conference, is strong on pharmacological and psychological treatments.

For shorter accounts see:

Clark, D.M. (1989) Anxiety states: panic and generalized anxiety. In: *Cognitive behaviour therapy for psychiatric problems: a practical guide* (eds K. Hawton, P. Salkovskis, J. Kirk and D.M. Clark), pp. 52–96. Oxford University Press, Oxford.

An authoritative account of cognitive-behavioural treatment.

Clark, D.M. (1997) Panic disorder and social phobia. In: *Science and practice of cognitive behaviour therapy* (eds D.M. Clark and C.G. Fairburn), pp. 121–153. Oxford University Press, Oxford.

Craske, M.G. and Lewin, M.R. (1998) Cognitive behavioural treatment of panic disorders. In: *International handbook of cognitive and behavioural treatments for psychological disorders* (ed. V.E. Caballo), pp. 105–28. Pergamon, Oxford.

A clear account of cognitive-behavioural treatment.

Non-technical

Useful accounts, including practical advice, are found in the following:

Baker, R. (1995) *Understanding panic attacks and overcoming fear.* Lion Publishing, Oxford.

An easy-to-read guide, with useful practical advice.

Barlow, D.H. and Craske, M.G. (1989) *Mastery of your anxiety and panic.* Graywind, Albany, USA.

Explanations and advice by two acknowledged experts.

Ingham, C. (1993) *Panic attacks: what they are, why they happen, and what you can do about them.* Thorsons, London.

A readable and detailed guide, written by someone who has herself suffered from panic.

Seligman, M.E.P. (1994) *What you can change and what you can't.* Knopf, New York, USA.

Clear, balanced account of psychological problems and treatment, including a chapter on panic disorder.

Westbrook, D. and Rout, K. (1998) *Understanding panic.* Clinical Psychology Department, Warneford Hospital, Oxford.

A clearly written brief guide, with information and advice.

Rachman, S. and de Silva, P. (2009) *Obsessive-compulsive disorder: the facts,* 4th edn. Oxford University Press, Oxford.

For an account of a related anxiety disorder, in this Series.

Index

Page numbers in bold indicate the major entry in the text.